Acknowledgements

The programme of research into social care for people with HIV-AIDS upon which this report is based was funded by the Department of Health and the Social Work Group of the Scottish Education Department. However, any opinions expressed in this report are the responsibility of the authors.

Many thanks must go to Sue Hennessy for her patient and diligent editing and proof reading of this report and also to Paula Press for the typing of the manuscript.

The research was conducted at the Universities of Hull and York between 1988 and 1990. The HIV-AIDS research team consisted of:

In Hull:

Robert Chester, Jenny Dagg, David Robinson and Philip Tether.

In York:

Maggie Bustard, Roy Carr-Hill, Alan Maynard, Keith Tolley and Glennis Whyte.

The authors would like to acknowledge the funding support and continuing interest of departmental staff from the Department of Health and Scottish Education Department. They would also like to thank the staff of all the SSDs and SWDs and of education, housing, health, and environmental health departments for sparing the time to provide information and advice. The staff of voluntary and self help groups were particularly helpful in giving information and helping to recruit interviewers and people with HIV-AIDS. The interviewers themselves did their work with commitment, sensitivity and skill.

The main debt of gratitude is, of course, to those people living with HIV-AIDS and their carers who were willing to tell us about the impact of the condition and about various aspects of social care demand and supply.

Contents

1 Assessment of the Supply and Demand of HIV-AIDS Services:

Data Collection and Methods

2 Living with AIDS

3 Using Informal and Formal Social Care

4 Organisation and Costs of Service Components:

Applying the Social Care Supply Framework (SCSF)

5 Financing Social Care and Costing Patterns of Use

List of Tables

List of Figures

1 Assessment of the Supply and Demand of HIV-AIDS Services:

Data Collection and Methods

1.1 Introduction

The reforms of community care in the UK will create a market for social care in which the local authority care agent will be the 'guardian' of the service user. This agent will be the budget holder and negotiate with other providers, such as the voluntary sector, for the appropriate supply of social care and related services. A continued growth in the numbers with HIV infection in the UK and a further shift in the location of care from hospital to the community will have important consequences for the operation of the community care market. This report examines in detail the need for social care for HIV infected individuals by focusing on the issues affecting the demand for and supply of services in the community.

1.2 HIV-AIDS and Social Care

This report is the product of a two year study carried out between September 1988 and September 1990 by the universities of Hull and York with the aim of examining the implications of HIV infection for the demand for and provision of social care and support services. In a narrow sense social care services provided 'formally' cover residential care, day care, domiciliary care and client based services provided by specialists such as social workers and occupational therapists. These services are provided by local authority social service departments, voluntary and private agencies. A wider scope for social care includes that provided 'informally' by relatives, partners and friends.

However, it is important to place the demand for and supply of such services within the context of the range of related services and support available to the individual. People with HIV infection will intermittently require health care (provided by health authorities/boards) and may also create a new demand for 'social services' such as housing, leisure, employment, education and social security (Figure 1). In addition, the existence of the virus has resulted in a need for statutory and voluntary agencies to provide health education and prevention initiatives related to HIV, which are generally based in the community.

Figure 1 Service Needs of People with HIV/AIDS.

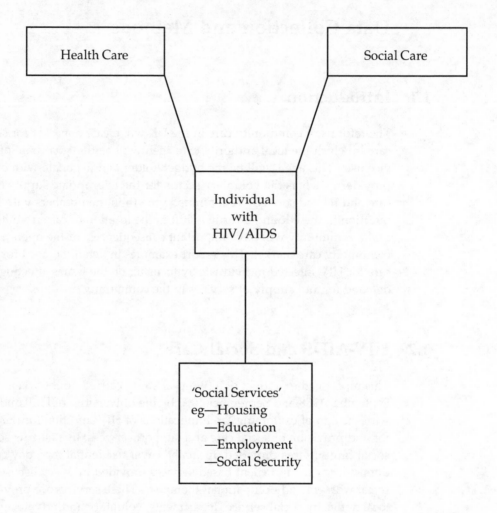

The demand for health care by each individual with HIV infection is
affected by the response of service providers to treating people with the
virus. For example, dentists' and general practitioners' attitudes towards the
virus is likely to affect the type of service they offer to HIV infected
individuals. The demand for social care and other local authority services
such as housing and employment is linked to the impact of the virus on the
daily lives of HIV+ individuals and their carers and the personal social and
economic circumstances facing individuals with the virus. The virus can
affect many facets of daily life, eg the appropriateness of existing

accommodation, the ability to undertake domestic tasks such as cooking and cleaning, participation in social activities, employment participation and income and the type of food consumed.

The supply of social and health care services in the community may not be closely related to the demand or need for care. This is due to a lack of information on demand patterns and unmet need (and hence a major reason for the research described in this report) and also because of political, organisational and resource constraints on the appropriate and effective provision of HIV-AIDS services. Such constraints have an important effect on the supply of social care, prevention services and social services (as defined in Figure 1). However, constraints on the supply of some health care may be associated with the social impact of the virus, and have also been examined in this study.

Specifically, the study had four main objectives:

1   To assess the personal social and financial impact of living with HIV infection.

2   To assess the social care and community health care service use (provided formally and informally), unmet demand and service needs of people with HIV infection, AIDS Related Complex (ARC) or AIDS and an examination of service quality and satisfaction.

3   To assess HIV-AIDS related social service organisation, policy, financing and funding and patterns of service supply.

4   To assess the costs of the demand for and supply of HIV-AIDS related social care services.

1.3   A Demand and Supply Framework

These objectives were addressed within a framework focusing on analysis of the demand and supply of HIV-AIDS services. The achievement of the first two objectives involved an analysis of the demand for HIV-AIDS services in the community. Although the focus was on social care, the participation in a survey conducted as part of the study of individuals across the range of stages of HIV infection provided a unique opportunity to examine differences in the demand for health care services, in particular that provided as part of a package of social and health care in the community. An assessment of unmet demand proved very difficult and consequently this report focuses on an examination of actual service use.

The achievement of the third aim required a detailed assessment of the supply of HIV-AIDS services by local authorities, in particular those services provided by Social Service Departments (SSDs) in England and Wales and Social Work Departments (SWDs) in Scotland, voluntary agencies and other providers of social services. This covered the supply of social care services for people affected by HIV infection (ie people with the virus, family, partners and others), HIV health education and prevention services, housing and accommodation services, advice/support services, the training of staff/volunteers (eg HIV awareness courses) and the use of resources for HIV-AIDS service monitoring and management/administration.

The assessment of the supply side role of Health Authorities and Health Boards was limited to examination of joint initiatives with local authorities and voluntary agencies in the organisation, provision and financing of health and social care. This covered two areas of work:

a) The direct provision of services such as hospital social work, hospital based occupational therapy, well-person clinics and community care support teams.

b) Jointly funded and managed HIV prevention initiatives such as needle exchanges or the provision of joint funding for voluntary agency initiatives (eg a new drug user centre in Edinburgh).

The analysis that was carried out to achieve the fourth objective involved both supply and demand side assessments. The analysis of resource use, funding and budget arrangements and costs of the supply of HIV-AIDS related services of three sets of agencies was examined. These were:

- Local authority Social Work Departments and Social Service Departments.

- Other local authority departments, in particular housing and education departments.

- Voluntary agencies involved in HIV-AIDS service provision.

Within each group of suppliers, variations in the use of specialist and non-specialist resources and costs for HIV-AIDS service delivery were examined.

4

Specialist resources covered staff such as HIV Coordinators and HIV-AIDS community care teams, budgets dedicated to providing a service for HIV-AIDS related purposes and services supplied by HIV-AIDS voluntary agencies such as the Terrence Higgins Trust and London Lighthouse. Non-specialist resources covered the use of existing staff and facilities for providing an HIV-AIDS service, such as SSD/SWD home helps, non-HIV specific voluntary agencies such as the Citizens Advice Bureau and general budgets for the provision of equipment for people with disabilities.

The supply side analysis was complemented by an analysis of the costs of meeting the demand for social care services by people with the virus. Five areas of service provided by SSD/SWDs, voluntary agencies, informal carers (family, friends, partners) and from the private sector were covered by the costing exercise:

- social worker services (hospital and community social workers)

- home support services (domiciliary care, volunteers, informal carers)

- practical goods and services (meals at home, occupational therapy, grants for specific items, domestic equipment, travel passes, private domestic services, home adaptions).

- health maintenance services (eg medication, massage)

- practical advice and emotional support (sexual, incontinence, diet and housing advice, telephone helplines).

1.4 The Study Localities

Detailed data collection on the demand for and supply of HIV-AIDS services was conducted in selected study localities in England and Scotland. On the supply side, an in-depth analysis was undertaken of HIV-AIDS service delivery policy and patterns of five local authorities: Hammersmith and Fulham, Kensington and Chelsea, Westminster (all London), Lothian (Scotland) and Manchester. These were selected according to known high numbers of HIV positive residents in the locality and/or where the local authority had established a strategy and pattern of service provision for HIV-AIDS.

Although data collection relating to voluntary agency service delivery and costs was centred around the five study localities agencies from outside the boundaries were also included to provide a more comprehensive picture of service supply. Voluntary agencies involved in HIV-AIDS related work varied from small local agencies such as the Leith Community Drugs Project to large organisations with a national catchment such as the Terrence Higgins Trust. In London in particular there is a greater likelihood of HIV positive individuals using the services of voluntary agencies located outside of the boundaries of the local authority in which they are a resident.

On the demand side, the five study localities provided the basis for the survey of the impact of the virus on individuals daily living and their social and health care service use and for a small survey covering informal carers. However, in order to increase the sample size further it was decided to also include individuals with the virus from other localities—the rest of Scotland (in particular Dundee and Glasgow), London (outside of the study areas) and Birmingham.

1.5 The Analysis of HIV-AIDS Service Demand and Supply

The Demand Study

The demand side study consisted of a detailed questionnaire based survey of people with HIV-AIDS.

The questionnaire was designed to collect data for two main subject areas:

i) **The socio-economic characteristics of individuals with the virus and the impact of the virus on their daily lives.**

Basic data was collected for each respondent on stage of infection (HIV+, ARC or AIDS), health status, location of residence, sex, age, living unit and composition, marital/partner situation, family, health status, accommodation and household amenities, education, employment status and income.

Data collection relating to the impact of the virus on daily life covered a number of specific topics:

- the antibody test and pre/post counselling provided
- illicit drug use

6

- the reactions of partners, relatives, friends and others to the individual revealing their HIV status.

- the medications (prescribed and non-prescribed) used by people with HIV infection to enhance their health.

- changes in smoking, alcohol and dietary behaviour and the use of 'alternative' therapies.

- changes in sexual behaviour.

- impact on accessibility and adequacy of housing and the need for specific household amenities or items.

- practical assistance required at home and use of social service home helps.

- transport and mobility difficulties experienced due to HIV infection and assistance from statutory providers.

- changes in employment and difficulties experienced at work.

- participation in voluntary work.

- the personal financial impact of the virus—this covered the personal cost of lost earnings and changes in expenditures on household items, food, health goods and sex products, alcohol consumption, regular household bills and leisure/social activities.

The primary method used to determine the impact of the virus on daily life was to ask individuals whether they had experienced any change in each of the areas covered since they had known they were HIV positive. The personal financial impact of employment changes due to the virus was derived by making various assumptions about the total loss of earnings over the previous two years from having time off work or becoming unemployed due to the virus. In addition, an estimate of the change in average weekly expenditures was calculated from the data provided in the questionnaire for each of the other items covered.

ii) **The use of social and health care services due to having the virus**. Data was collected for several areas of service use:

- the use of antibody testing services and counselling services.

- the use of informal care for practical assistance and emotional support, and help provided for carers.

- the use of the voluntary and self-help sector eg HIV specific, national organisations, drug agencies.

- the use of social services ie social workers,

- the use of health services ie outpatient, inpatient, home care, primary care, dental services.

- the use of private services ie for practical assistance, special products and private health insurance/treatment.

In addition to data on service use respondents were asked questions relating to service quality, the satisfaction with service provision, attitudes towards the service provided and their perceived care needs.

Respondents were also asked to complete two sets of diaries over a seven day period following interview:

a) A 'care diary' covering all the help received from health and social service specialists (eg consultants, GP, home helps, family care assistants), voluntary organisations (eg helpline, Body Positive, drugs groups) and friends, family and partners. Information was requested on whether the help was received at home, the time of arrival, the length of visit and type of help provided.

b) A 'financial diary' listing detailed expenditures incurred each day. However, the only data that proved useful from this exercise was that for expenditures on diet which was included in the assessment of the personal financial impact of the virus.

Invitations to participate in the survey were distributed through local voluntary and self-help groups. The invitations consisted of a 'pack' containing a covering letter, a short project outline and a consent form. This was an 'opportunistic' approach designed to reach not only those people in contact with statutory health and social services but also those whose only source of social care was the non-statutory sector. In addition, respondents were recruited via advertisements in the Body Positive and Frontliners newsletter and from 'packs' distributed by the Genito-Urinary Medicine (GUM) clinic at the West London Hospital. The recruitment role of 'key workers' and other interviewers was particularly important in Manchester and Lothian where it was difficult to gain the wholehearted cooperation of the voluntary agencies.

Once an individual with HIV infection had agreed to participate in the survey a meeting was arranged with a trained interviewer/key worker to complete the questionnaire. A team of paid interviewers were recruited for each of the study localities mainly through HIV specific voluntary agencies. Most interviews took between two and six hours depending on the circumstances for the interview and the health of the respondent. On completion of the interview respondents were asked whether they would complete a care and financial diary, their availability for re-interview and for consent to contact a main informal carer as identified by the respondent.

Targets were originally set for the recruitment of HIV+, ARC and AIDS respondents in each of the study areas. These were 150 respondents in the London area and 50 each in Manchester and Lothian. Once it became obvious that these targets were too ambitious it was decided to include individuals from Birmingham and other parts of Scotland who had been identified by key workers as willing to participate in the survey. In total 181 first interviews were carried out over a 15 month period from January 1989 to March 1990 (Table 1.1). Because of the slow and difficult process involved in accumulating the sample only 46 re-interviews were possible covering those respondents originally seen earliest. Also limited success was achieved with the informal carer interview and care and financial diaries. A questionnaire was designed to ask informal carers about their care role and the support they received and required. However, only 25 informal carers were identified by respondents and of these only 14 could be interviewed. A total of 18 financial diaries and 49 care diaries were completed (Table 1.1).

Table 1.1 **Questionnaire Interviews Carried Out and Diary Returns**

	First Interviews	Re- Interviews	Carer Interviews	Financial Diaries	Care Diaries
London	81	26	8	14	30
Manchester	48	20	4	4	8
Lothian	33	—	2	—	7
Birmingham	19	—	—	—	4
Total	181	46	14	18	49

Data analysis was conducted for the sample of 181 individuals with HIV infection. This analysis was conducted at the level of the complete sample, or disaggregated according to the stage of HIV infection (HIV+, ARC, AIDS) and the locality of the respondents.

Several lessons were learnt from the use of opportunistic methods to recruit HIV positive individuals to the survey and the design of interview led questionnaire surveys for such individuals. The approach provided a number of important benefits:

- a flexibility to enable recruitment of individuals across the range of HIV+, ARC and AIDS who were using a wide variety of social and community health care services.

- high quality of the completed questionnaires because of the skill of the trained interviewers and a well-designed format.

- useful information on the characteristics of HIV+ individuals, the impact of the virus on lifestyle and social and health care service use and needs.

- significant cooperation and involvement of the HIV voluntary sector in promoting the research project.

However, the approach and questionnaire design demonstrated a number of important problems:

- a poor response from the distribution of invitation 'packs' to the voluntary agencies. It appeared that they gave only low priority to their distribution despite constant reminders, including visits from team members. More success was achieved from the advertisements in the Body Positive and Frontliners newsletters and the active promotion of the project by clinicians at the West London Hospital GUM clinic. These sources yielded 76 per cent (62) of all the London respondents.

- because of the nature of the recruitment there was a tendency towards a high use of voluntary services among the participants. This bias was partially offset by the recruitment through the GUM clinic in London. The sample did not represent a scientifically controlled selection, which was, however, virtually impossible to achieve for a survey of social care for HIV infected individuals.

- the questionnaire proved most difficult to use with intravenous drug users because of its length and a relatively limited attention time span of these respondents. In several cases drug users completing the interview were allowed to 'talk freely' in relation to a number of topics in the questionnaire with attempts made subsequently to fit their response to the specific questions in the questionnaire.

The questionnaire represented a pragmatic cross-sectional approach to the collection of data on HIV impact and service use of individuals with the virus. This involved a 'before and after' method by which respondents were asked to recall changes related to having the virus. Whilst this study design lacks scientific rigour, it was a practical approach to providing an overview of impact, social and health care service use and needs associated with living with the virus.

The Analysis of Service Supply

The analysis of service supply involved the collection of data on HIV-AIDS service organisation, resource use and type of services provided by the statutory and voluntary sector in the study localities.

Data was collected from statutory service providers by two main means:

i) A series of semi-structured interviews with key managers in the SSD/SWD, senior personnel in other local authority departments and AIDS Coordinators in health districts providing services within the five localities.

ii) A self-administered questionnaire which was sent to team leaders of specific social service providers in the five localities.

SSD/SWD managers included HIV-AIDS Coordinators, Divisional and Assistant Divisional Directors, Principal Officers responsible for major areas of social work provision and 'HIV- specialist' posts of all kinds. Care was taken to ensure that the experiences and views of Housing Departments and Environmental Health Departments in the five localities were obtained. A total of 47 interviews were conducted and the material from these was discussed at length with AIDS Coordinators in the relevant health authorities.

The data from the interviews and related policy documents enabled a detailed examination of the HIV-AIDS service organisation/policy of the study local authorities, their service strategies and provision in 1989/90 and plans for future service development.

Self-administered questionnaires were sent to four groups of social service providers: domiciliary care managers (for home help teams), and team leaders for occupational therapy, hospital social work and area social work. Information was requested on the staffing resources available, the skill-mix of the team, the existence of HIV-AIDS specialists in the team, the type of service provided and the HIV-AIDS client group served, HIV related training received by members of the team and the views of the team leader/manager as to the most important HIV-AIDS related work issues they and other service providers face.

The number of questionnaires sent out/returned is shown in Table 1.2.

Table 1.2   **Occupational Groups Questionnaire Response**

	London Boroughs		Manchester		Lothian	
Domiciliary Care	12	(n=48)	17	(n=39)	16	(n=19)
OTs	5	(n=15)	0	(n=0)	11	(n=18)
Hospital Social Work	18	(n=39)	5	(n=6)	2	(n=6)
Area Social Work Team Leaders[1]	36	(n=52)	42	(n=59)	8	(n=18)[2]
Other[3]	12	(n=38)	0	(n=7)	7	(n=6)

[1] In Manchester—Health Teams

[2] Returns from Team Managers cover adult, mental handicap, emergency duty and family support workers.

[3] 'Other' covers Children's Services Education Officers, Residential Officers and community Drugs Team Workers.

Voluntary organisations in each of the five localities provided a wide range of social care services to people with HIV infection and AIDS, and to their informal carers. The contribution of both 'AIDS-specific' and 'non-AIDS-specific' voluntary organisations to the provision of social care was sought in two ways.

i)   A self-administered questionnaire seeking information on the provision of social care services, sources of funding, staffing, liaison and cooperation between voluntary agencies and with statutory organisations, plans for the future, and involvement in other HIV-related areas of work such as prevention and education. This was sent to 57 AIDS-specific organisations (including London and nationwide groups) and a sample of 275 non-AIDS-specific organisations across the study localities.

ii) Semi-structured interviews with key informants within regional and national AIDS-specific organisations were carried out. The interview discussion included the range of services provided by these groups, funding, monitoring and evaluation, staffing, coordination arrangements both between voluntary agencies and with the statutory sector, and plans for the future.

A total of 332 voluntary organisations active in the five authorities were invited to complete the self-administered questionnaire. Table 1.3 provides details of the returns.

Table 1.3   **Voluntary Agency Survey—Response**

	AIDS Specific		Non-AIDS Specific	
London/National	17	(n=38)	31	(n=94)
Manchester	2	(n=6)	6	(n=83)
Lothian	8	(n=13)	38	(n=98)
TOTAL	**27**	**(n=57)**	**75**	**(n=275)**

The overall response rate was 31 per cent. This masks both variations between AIDS and non-AIDS-specific groups (response rates of 47 and 27 per cent respectively), and between study areas—the response rate was much lower in Manchester (9 per cent) than in London (36 per cent) and Lothian (41 per cent). Thirteen respondents from key AIDS-specific organisations were interviewed. The information from questionnaires and interviews was supplemented by (i) the semi-structured interviews with AIDS Co-ordinators in the study localities and SSD voluntary organisation liaison officers and (ii) analysis of SSD policy documents, voluntary organisations' Annual Reports and other documents.

1.6   National Survey of SSD/SWDs

A national survey of SSDs and SWDs was conducted which provided information on the budgets developed by SSD/SWDs and other local authority departments in England, Scotland and Wales for HIV-AIDS services in 1988/89 and 1989/90. The size and structure of these budgets varied across authorities according to the number of HIV positive service users, the service strategy and the availability of Central Government AIDS Support Grant (in England). A total grant of £7 million was made available in 1989/90 and £10 million in 1990/91. The survey enabled a comparison between the budget arrangements for HIV-AIDS services in Scotland, where no ring fenced allocation was made by the Scottish Office, and that for England and Wales where 'special money' was allocated. In addition, an assessment was made of the specific HIV-AIDS budget arrangements adopted by the five study authorities.

The organisation of a national survey of SSD/SWDs involves several important stages. Prior to the survey, meetings were held between members of the project team and the Association of Directors of Social Services (ADSS)

Research Committee in respect of departments in England and Wales, and the Association of Directors of Social Work (ADSW) Research Sub-committee in respect of Scottish departments. Nominees from these two bodies were subsequently consulted regarding questionnaire design. With the approval of the ADSS and the ADSW, 123 social service and social work departments outside the five study localities, were circularised in March 1989 to explain the study, and copies of any policy documents regarding HIV-related service provision were requested.

In 1989 a structured questionnaire was forwarded to named contacts in 118 departments which had agreed to participate in the survey. A total of 65 SSD/SWDs completed the questionnaire. A breakdown of responses across local authorities is provided in Table 1.4.

Table 1.4   **National Survey of SSD/SWDs—Responses**

Local Authority Area	Number Received
London Boroughs	12
Metropolitan Districts	18
County Councils	28
Scottish Regions	7
	65

1.7   Evaluation of Costs

The evaluation of costs covered a supply and demand analysis. In the supply side assessment, the current annual costs of HIV-AIDS service supply of the five study authorities was examined. The distribution of costs across service organisation and resource use areas was identified using the Social Care Supply Framework (SCSF) which is described below. A variety of aggregate estimates were produced for actual one year costs, potential one year costs (ie if all resources, such as staff, had been available for a full 12 month period) and the costs of HIV-specialist resource use only.

The calculation of the aggregate costs of the supply of HIV-AIDS services by the five study authorities involved estimation of the use of staff resources, the provision of equipment and grants to people with HIV infection or

AIDS, other non-staff costs such as travel, postage, stationery, central organisation overheads (eg central management and support services, administration), and premise use. Data for the costing was derived from all sources used in the supply side study. For example, estimates of the time of SSD/SWD social workers spent on specific HIV-AIDS related activities were derived from the questionnaires completed by social work team leaders. Estimates of the unit costs of each resource were derived from several sources. As an illustration, actual staff salaries or mid-points (if the specific grade of staff providing a service was not known) for 1989/90 were used to calculate the costs of staff resources. The costs of specialist HIV staff resources were costed using a different formula from that for non-specialist resources to reflect the greater level of management and administrative support required for the HIV related work of the former. A detailed description of the supply side costing methodology is available from the authors at the Centre for Health Economics at York University.

In addition, an assessment of the annual costs of the service supplied by a sample of HIV specific and drug related voluntary agencies in the five study localities was undertaken. Costs were calculated for 36 agencies who had returned a financial statement covering at least one year between 1987–91 and/or provided resource use data on a completed voluntary agency questionnaire. Costs were calculated for the use of paid staff, non-staff costs and estimated volunteer time.

This supply side analysis produced aggregate costs of total service provision. This was complemented by a detailed assessment of the case-specific costs of social care service use by people with HIV infection or AIDS in order to determine the average cost of the current demand for care. Specific details of the costing methodology are provided in chapter 5.4.

1.8 The Social Care Supply Framework (SCSF)—a planning and accounting framework

A framework was developed to examine the organisation and structure of HIV-AIDS service supply and to assess the resources directed to several areas of service provision. This social care supply framework (SCSF) can be applied to assess the HIV-AIDS related service provision of local authorities and other agencies. It represents a versatile method of examining the balance of resource use in HIV-AIDS service provision and for determining what is spent, what could be spent and what is needed to meet all service demands.

The SCSF consists of six key components, which combine to produce a total local authority service supply (SS). The framework has the following structure:

SS = MC + T + PE + H + SC + ME

where SS = service supply, MC = service management and co-ordination, T = training, PE = HIV related prevention and health education, H = housing, SC = direct social care and support, ME = monitoring and evaluation. The framework can be extended to incorporate service supply by the voluntary sector (+ V) and by informal carers (+ IC).

This framework was developed from the experiences of HIV-AIDS service provision within the five high profile authorities who participated in the study. The objective was to use it to assess local authority involvement in HIV-AIDS services from two inter-related perspectives:

a) the key organisational/policy issues involved in local authority HIV-AIDS service supply

b) the distribution of costs to the local authority of providing an HIV-AIDS related service.

1.9 The Structure of the Report

The central focus for the assessment of supply and demand was in the delivery and use of social care services such as social worker services, domiciliary care, occupational therapy, day centres and other practical and emotional support.

The following chapters examine the relationship between the demand for and the provision of social care for people with HIV-AIDS. Chapter 2 provides an outline of the impact of HIV infection on the daily lives of individuals living with the virus and carers. The use of informal and formal social health care is examined in Chapter 3. The supply of HIV-AIDS social care services in five study authorities forms the focus of Chapter 4. This uses the SCSF to assess the distribution of costs across service activity categories.

Finally, Chapter 5 includes an assessment of the financing of social service/social work HIV-AIDS service development and estimates of the average cost per person of various packages of social care for people with HIV infection or AIDS.

2 Living with HIV-AIDS

The questionnaire-based survey of people with HIV-AIDS provided a wealth of material on the impact of the diagnosis on various aspects of everyday life including finances.

2.1 People with HIV-AIDS

Participation in the Survey

The recruitment procedure outlined in chapter 1 was designed to assemble a group of people ranging from those newly-diagnosed as HIV positive to those with well-established AIDS. The broad categorisation of the sample is presented in Table 2.1.

Table 2.1   **The Nature of the HIV-AIDS Sample**

Respondents' Characteristics	Number	Percentage of total sample
HIV positive only	106	59
ARC (pre AIDS, symptomatic HIV etc)	35	19
AIDS	40	22
	181	**100**

The Respondents

The background characteristics of the 181 respondents included, in brief:

gender; 93 per cent were men, with Scotland having the highest percentage of women (16 per cent)

age; ranged from 19–64 with 47 per cent clustered in the 26–35 age group. Of London respondents 37 per cent were over 40 compared with only 9 per cent in Scotland.

marital/family status; 61 per cent were single, 29 per cent had partners, including gay partners.

living unit; 52 per cent reported living alone, with Birmingham having the highest percentage (63 per cent) and Scotland the lowest (32 per cent).

education; 45 per cent of Scottish respondents had academic or professional qualifications; Manchester had the highest figure, 79 per cent.

money; Scottish respondents had the lowest income levels with 45 per cent earning less than £50 per week compared with 36 per cent in Manchester and 15 per cent in London.

Antibody Testing

All respondents in the survey had had their HIV status confirmed by antibody testing: 83 per cent at their local hospital, with very few using private clinics or general practitioners (5 per cent), although 16 per cent of the Scottish sample were tested by their GP due mainly to their presenting simultaneously with problems concerned with drug use. The main reason for seeking a test was the general suspicion of having the virus because of current or past sexual or drug-related activity (60 per cent) and/or because of the onset of ill health (48 per cent). However, 9 per cent stated that they had sought a test to confirm that they did not have the virus.

There were a number of people (14 per cent) who did not know they were being tested and who, therefore, received no pre-test counselling. In addition, a further 47 per cent of the sample had no pre-test counselling. The data given in table 2.2 suggest that the availability of such counselling

Table 2.2   **Pre-Test Counselling Received**

Year of Diagnosis	Pre-test counselling:		No pre-test counselling:	
	Number	percentage	Number	percentage
1983	—	—	3	100
1984	3	23	10	77
1985	8	21	30	79
1986	11	34	21	66
1987	14	39	22	61
1988	20	54	17	46
1989	14	67	7	33
1990	—	—	1	100

Table 2.3 **Post-test Counselling Received**

Year of Diagnosis	Pre-test counselling:		No pre-test counselling:	
	Number	percentage	Number	percentage
1983	3	100	—	—
1984	8	62	5	38
1985	20	53	18	47
1986	20	63	12	37
1987	20	56	1	44
1988	25	68	12	32
1989	15	71	6	29
1990	1	100	—	—

has increased over time: 23 per cent of those tested in 1984 received counselling whereas by 1989 the figure had risen to 67 per cent. As far as post-
test counselling is concerned 38 per cent of the sample received none (Table
2.3). Half of those people who had been tested without their knowledge
received neither pre- nor post-test counselling.

The data in Table 2.4 show the year of initial diagnosis. People with HIV-
AIDS may be diagnosed as having the virus weeks, months or years following seroconversion and therefore these data do not indicate the duration of
infection for this sample which is unknown. The earliest recorded diagnosis
for this sample was 1983 (three people) and the most recent was 1990 (one
person).

Table 2.4 **Year of Initial Diagnosis**

Year	Number	% of Total
1983	3	1.7
1984	13	7.2
1985	38	21.0
1986	32	17.7
1987	36	19.9
1988	37	20.4
1989	21	11.6
1990	1	0.5
Total	**181**	**100.0**

The following table shows the year of initial diagnosis by the respondents' current HIV status. As noted above, the duration of infection is unknown as is the duration of current diagnosis. However, the data show a number of people who have not deteriorated to ARC or AIDS since an original diagnosis as HIV positive.

Table 2.5 **Year of Initial Diagnosis and Current HIV Status**

	HIV Positive (n=106)		ARC (n=35)		AIDS (n=40)	
	No.	% HIV	No.	HIV	No.	ARC
1983	2	2	1	3	—	—
1984	8	7	—	—	5	12.5
1985	18	17	10	28	10	25
1986	19	18	17	20	6	15
1987	20	19	11	31	5	12.5
1988	22	21	3	9	12	30
1989	16	15	3	9	2	5
1990	1	1	—	—	—	—
Total	106	100	35	100	40	100

Health status

A number of questions were asked concerning health status:

i) a self-assessment of health state at the time of the interview;

ii) experience of HIV-related physical and psychological health problems;

iii) experience of existing long-standing conditions prior to diagnosis.

Although only nine people (5 per cent) reported having experienced no apparent symptoms, 71 (39 per cent) stated that their health at the time of the interview was 'good' or 'excellent'. When these data are examined by HIV status they show that people with ARC and AIDS assessed their health as 'poor' or 'very poor' more frequently than people who were HIV positive only.

Table 2.6 Self-Assessment of Health Status

	Number	% of Total
Very poor	11	6
Poor	35	19
Fair	62	34
Good	58	32
Excellent	13	7
Not known	2	1
Total	**181**	**100**

Table 2.7 Self-Assessment of Health by HIV Status

	HIV POS (n=106)		ARC (n=35)		AIDS (n=40)	
	No.	% HIV POS	No.	% ARC	No.	% AIDS
Very poor	2	2	4	11	5	12
Poor	15	14	6	17	14	35
Fair	27	25	19	54	16	40
Good	51	48	4	11	3	8
Excellent	10	9	2	6	1	2
Not known	1	1	—	—	1	2

Health Problems

When asked what health problems they had experienced since knowing that they had the virus, 172 respondents (95 per cent) reported having experienced at least one of the range of health problems and 72 per cent had experienced more than one. These data refer to the respondent's own opinion as to their health state and no attempt was made to evaluate statements diagnostically, although respondents were asked both for their experience of illness and the effect (physical or psychological) of having that illness. In certain instances, the differentiation between 'illness' and 'effect' is difficult to determine. For example, where respondents cited 'depression' or 'anxiety' as an outcome of having the virus, it is not possible to state with certainty whether this refers to clincial depression and psychological illness, or a symptom/effect of other conditions or other social factors. Similarly, 'fatigue' may, for example, be a symptom of persistent generalised lymphadenopathy, the effect of other clinical conditions; or the outcome of stress. The most frequently cited problems are shown in Table 2.8.

Table 2.8   **Most Frequently Cited Health Problems**

	Number	% of People with Health Problems (n=172)	% of Total Sample (n=181)
Depression/anxiety	91	53	50
Candida	53	31	29
Weakness/fatigue	37	22	20
Pneumocystis Carinii Pneumonia (PCP)	24	14	13
Non specific skin infections	19	11	10
Weight loss	19	11	10
No specific respiratory infection	18	10	10
Night-sweats	17	10	9
Diarrhoea	15	9	8

In addition to those people citing depression or anxiety as a health outcome from having the virus, 124 (69 per cent) stated that they had experienced phases of acute or chronic depression as an effect of having other conditions, often because each new illness or recurring bout of illness was interpreted by the individual as a further deterioration of the immune system and a possible indicator of AIDS.

Everyone was asked whether they were registered, for example with local authorities, in respect of physical and sensory impairment. Registration may have taken place prior to HIV infection due to pre-existing disablement. The results are shown in Table 2.9.

Table 2.9   **Registration for Impairment by HIV Status**

	HIV+ (n=106)	ARC (n=35)	AIDS (n=40)	Total (n=181)
Disabled	9%	29%	35%	18%
Chronically sick	6%	11%	35%	13%
Hearing impaired	*	—	*	1%
Speech impaired	*	—	—	*
Sight impaired	2%	6%	3%	3%

* = 1 person

Illicit Drug Use

The survey did not ask whether respondents were aware of how they had contracted the virus and in respect of drug use the method of usage was not always reported—therefore the extent of past or present drug use cannot be taken as an indicator of routes of infection. Respondents were asked whether, apart from medications, they used drugs on a regular basis currently or had done so in the past few years. Forty respondents (22 per cent) stated that they were ex or current drug users. Their use varied from the occasional 'recreational' use to the habitual. Substances included cannabis, nitrites and hallucinogens and other stimulants. In some cases, people use a combination of so-called 'hard' and 'soft' drugs. Where recreational or habitual drug use was reported, it was rare for respondents to use one drug solely. Table 2.10 sets out the different substances used. This almost certainly understates the extent of use as some drug users provided few details of specific substances or stated that they used 'whatever was available'.

The reported changes in drug use since diagnosis were often complex in that whilst a number of people had stopped using drugs or substances altogether, others had changed the type of substance used, such as ceasing to use 'hard' drugs in favour of 'soft' drugs, or had changed their methods of using, such as no longer injecting. Those who were on prescribed maintenance programmes (methadone) had, ostensibly, ceased certain forms of drug use but it was clear from a number of interviews that some respondents 'topped up' their methadone prescription with other substances. The extent of 'prescription' drug use (eg, temgesic, DF118, and tranquillisers) is complicated by the fact that a number of ex and current drug users received such drugs legally because of symptoms related to HIV or withdrawal.

Table 2.10   **The Type of Drugs and Substances Used**

Drug	No. of Users
Heroin (IV–18, non-IV–3)	21
Cannabis	17
LSD	10
Amphetamines (IV–1, non-IV–8)	9
Benzodiazepines	9
Cocaine (IV–1, non-IV–5)	6
Diconal/DF118/Temgesic	6
Nitrites	5
Barbiturates	4
'Ecstacy'	4
Opium/morphine	2

When respondents used substances for recreational use or only occasionally they often did not consider their use of such substances to be a problem in terms of needing to stop or requiring any services or support. The use of cannabis was frequently cited by respondents as a 'positive' aid to relaxation and stress reduction. Bearing in mind the difficulty in assessing change in drug use, the following data (Table 2.11) show the reported changes in drug and substance use since the respondents have known their HIV status:

Table 2.11   **Reported Changes in Drug Use Since HIV Diagnosis**

	No Use	Less Use	Different Use[1]	More Use	No change
'Recreational' drugs/substances	5	2	—	1	4
Non-'recreational' drugs/substances	12	4	5	2	3
Total	17	6	5	3	9
Percentage of total responses %	43	15	12	7	23

[1] For example 'no longer inject', 'no longer share equipment', 'share equipment less', 'use different drugs' etc.

2.2 Revealing HIV Status and Maintaining Health

Maintaining health after diagnosis of HIV infection can take many forms. It is also closely related to the willingness to reveal the diagnosis to family, friends and others.

Revealing HIV Status

In order to assess the extent of confidentiality and also the availability of networks of informal support, respondents were asked whether certain people or service providers had been informed of their HIV status and how that information had been revealed. It is clear that people with the virus make careful decisions about who they inform of their HIV status—not only to avoid potentially hostile reactions but also to avoid causing distress to others.

Seventeen people had told none of their personal contacts of their HIV status and the most frequent reason for this was that the respondent feared rejection. The following data refer therefore to the remaining 163 respondents who had decided to inform one or more of their personal contacts of their status.

A total of 339 contacts were reported. Table 2.12 shows the category of people told and their reaction to the news. The 'reactions' have been categorised as follows:

Supportive: the person, whilst undoubtedly upset and anxious, was nevertheless understanding and helpful to the respondent.

Unsupportive: the person rejected the respondent, for example, refused further contact or exhibited hostility towards the respondent.

Distressed: the person was distressed to the point of being unable to discuss the issue, exhibiting features of shock or denial.

Other: for example, where the person had not been informed by the respondent him/herself and the reaction was unknown.

Responses confirmed that the respondents were highly selective in their choice of whom to inform of their HIV status. As Table 2.12 shows, a number of friends and family members found the news too traumatic to be able

Table 2.12   **People Informed of HIV Status and their Reaction**

	Percentage of all contacts		Percentage of Contacts:			
			Supportive	Unsupportive	Distressed	Other
Friends	42	(n=143)	74	11	11	4
Parent(s)	21	(n=71)	48	8	20	24
Partner & ex-partners	20	(n=66)	74	11	14	1
Siblings	14	(n=48)	62	4	17	17
Other relatives	3	(n=11)	73	—	18	9

to offer support and the respondents' concern to avoid causing such distress was a frequent reason for their not informing others. Additionally, many respondents felt that their HIV status should not be revealed until such a time as disclosure was absolutely necessary, for example, if they became terminally ill. The feeling was that 'there is no point in upsetting 'x' now . . .'.

Table 2.13 shows the percentage of informal contacts who were not told of the person's HIV status and the reasons for this decision. A total of 146 contacts were reported. The categories of reasons are as follows:

Upsetting: providing the information would be too upsetting either for the respondent or the recipient of the news.

Deferring the Decision: not wishing to inform/upset someone until 'necessary', eg, serious or terminal illness.

Rejection: fear of rejection or hostility.

No point: the respondent is not sufficiently 'close' to the relative/friend: little contact or communication: '[they] would not understand'.

Lifestyle: informing the person would provoke questions about or revelation of the respondents' sexuality/ drug use etc.

Other: includes fears concerning breaches of confidentiality, unspecified reasons etc.

Table 2.13   **People Not Informed of HIV Status and Reasons**

	Percentage of all contacts		Percentage of Contacts					
			Upsetting	Deferring the Decision	Rejection	No point	Life Style	Other
Parent(s)	44	(n=65)	32	25	12	15	9	6
Friends	28	(n=41)	5	5	54	22	2	12
Other relatives	15	(n=22)	9	—	14	45	9	23
Siblings	8	(n=11)	18	36	—	27	9	9
Partners & ex-partners	5	(n=7)	29	14	43	—	—	14
	100	**146**						

Prescribed Medication

Only 30 respondents (17 per cent) in this sample of people with HIV, ARC or AIDS were not taking prescribed medication at the time of the interview. The use of prescribed medication amongst the remaining 151 respondents was high as can be seen in Table 2.14. Data were collected on the type of medication prescribed, the frequency of prescriptions, what the medication was for and the financial cost to the individual, if any. The impact of taking any drug or medication will be felt mainly in respect of its effectiveness in preventing, controlling or curing symptoms or conditions. A secondary impact may be in respect of any physical side-effects of drug or other treatment, for example, the possible side-effects of taking AZT or receiving chemotherapy.

Some medications had been used during a particular period of illness or for a particular symptom and then stopped but the majority of items mentioned by respondents were in current use, with the frequency of prescriptions ranging from every week to every two months. The majority of respondents were taking more than one form of medication. Table 2.14 shows the number of items taken by respondents in respect of their HIV status.

The ten most frequently prescribed items are shown in Table 2.15.

Table 2.14   **Prescribed Medications**

Number of Medications	Number of Respondents	Percentage of sample (n=181)
0	30	17
1	39	22
2	18	10
3	48	27
4	13	7
5	15	8
6	4	2
7	6	3
8	8	8
	181	100

Table 2.15   **Most Frequently Prescribed Medications**

Name	Number of Respondents[1]	Percentage of Sample (n=181)
AZT	94	52
Acyclovir	44	24
Fluconazole	32	18
Pentamidine	22	12
Antibiotics (unspecified)	19	10
Septrin	14	8
Temazapan	14	8
Diazepam	14	8
Methadone	14	8
Hydrocortisone	11	6

[1] respondents often took more than one medication.

In addition to using prescribed medications 83 respondents (46 per cent of the sample) made virus-related purchases from chemists, herbalists, health-food shops. There were, however, regional differences in purchasing as Table 2.16 shows:

Table 2.16 **Purchase of Non-Prescribed Items**

	Total	London	Manchester	Scotland
Number	83	52	16	15
Percentage	46	64	24	48

Forty separate items were mentioned. The most requent were vitamins and minerals (73 purchases) and other popular items included:

- skin creams
- evening primrose oil
- royal jelly
- cod liver oil
- dietary supplements eg, Complan
- yoghurt (for candida)
- herbal preparations/tonics
- antiseptics and disinfectants.

Smoking

A high percentage of respondents (66 per cent) said that they were smokers prior to knowing that they had the virus. A further six respondents said that they were ex-smokers at the time of diagnosis. As Table 2.17 shows, this figure for smoking prevalence is approximately twice as high as that for the general population (OPCS, 1990).

Table 2.17 **Smoking Prevalence prior to HIV knowledge by Age: Sample and National Data**

Age Group	Sample: % of age group	National: % of age group
20–24	76	37
25–34	67	36
35–49	64	36
50–59	54	33
All age groups	66	32

There was evidence of an overall reduction in the average tobacco consumption of respondents since having the virus. In most cases, however, people did not change their tobacco consumption levels. It was found that overall 61 per cent (n=111) of the respondents were cigarette, pipe or cigar smokers at the time of the interview. This was marginally less than the proportion who had smoked tobacco prior to having the virus.

Alcohol

The great majority of people in the sample stated that they drank alcohol prior to their original diagnosis: all thirteen of the women and 147 men (88 per cent) of the men.

Ninety six respondents (60 per cent) who drank alcohol, stated that they had changed their pattern of drinking since knowing that they had the virus.

Table 2.18　**Changes in Alcohol Consumption since Diagnosis**

Change	Men		Women		Total	
	No.	% of all men in survey	No.	% of all women in survey	No.	% of total sample
Stopped	14	10	5	38	19	10
Drink less	56	38	2	15	58	32
Drink more	16	11	3	23	19	10

Food

A series of questions concerning respondents' eating patterns were included in this survey to assess:

i)　the extent of awareness of health eating
ii)　the dietary advice received and from whom
iii)　the changes, if any, in dietary habits since being diagnosed
iv)　any changes in spending on food.

The importance of maintaining a healthy, balanced diet has been emphasised for people with HIV infection, particularly since symptoms such as severe weight loss, intestinal infections and mouth infections which deter eating are common. There is also the possibility of some people with HIV infection experiencing malabsorbtion due to the virus or infections of the gut.

Twenty four respondents (13 per cent of the sample) stated they followed a particular diet prior to knowing that they had the virus either out of preference, for example a vegetarian or macrobiotic diet, because of pre-existing health needs, for example diabetes, or because of their culture. Advice on diet had been received by 42 per cent of the sample, most usually from a dietician but sometimes from health professionals or voluntary organisations. A higher proportion (53 per cent) of people with ARC or AIDS had received such advice compared with people who were HIV positive.

The nature of the advice received was based, generally, on the recommendation to eat more fresh produce—fruit and vegetables—and to increase protein input. But there were variations which may have resulted from a need to tailor dietary advice to an individual's personal health state or achievable goals. So, for example, some respondents were advised to avoid fats and sugars, to increase fibre intake, and to avoid pre-cooked or cook-chill foods.

Illness, and in particular conditions such as mouth infections or gastro-intestinal disorders, may inhibit appetite or deter people from eating. However, where dietary change occurred it was largely as a result of choice or economic necessity rather than illness. Dietary changes had been made by 117 respondents (65 per cent of the sample) since knowing that they had the virus.

A majority of respondents in each diagnostic group had made dietary changes and, as table 2.19 shows, people with ARC or AIDS had more frequently changed their diet.

Table 2.19   **Changes in Dietary Behaviour by Diagnosis**

HIV Positive	ARC	AIDS
59%	65%	75%

Changes in dietary behaviour could be 'positive' that is, eating more healthily, or 'negative' changes where respondents ate less well since diagnosis. The majority of respondents making changes adopted one or more 'positive' approaches to eating, for example:

- eating more of a recommended food, eg fruit, vegetables   60 respondents   33%

- eating a better 'balanced' or 'healthier' diet   54 respondents   30%

Some examples of 'negative' changes included: eating more 'junk' food and 'take-aways'; being unable to afford a 'proper' or recommended diet; and having no appetite.

These data on dietary habits were analysed to see whether respondents were more or less likely to have made changes following receipt of dietary advice (Table 2.20). While there is a relationship between the receipt of dietary advice and dietary change, in that 79 per cent of respondents receiving advice made changes, a high proportion (54 per cent) of people not receiving formal advice made changes also.

Table 2.20   **Advice and Dietary Changes**

	Percentage of those having advice (n=76)	Percentage of those not having advice (n=105)	Percentage of total sample (n=181)
Eating more regularly	51	40	44
Eating less regularly	21	23	22
Eating more food	37	25	30
Eating less food	32	28	29
Eating different diet	64	27	43
Percentage with dietary change	79	54	64

Eating less food can be either a positive change, for example, eating less but more healthier food, or a negative change, for example, not eating enough food to maintain a health diet. In fact, the majority of those people eating less food were doing so as a result of 'negative' dietary changes.

'Alternative' Therapies

In addition to making changes in dietary habits and purchasing items such as vitamins, herbal preparations and nutritional supplements, some respondents to this survey also used less orthodox therapies or treatments to promote their physical or psychological well-being, such as massage, acupuncture, reflexology, aromatherapy, and homeopathic treatments. Thirty three respondents (18 per cent of the sample) had used such treatments via a voluntary or self-help organisation and 28 respondents (15 per cent of the sample) had used private treatments.

Sexual Behaviour

Because the human immunodeficiency virus can be transmitted through sexual behaviour, it is necessary to consider also the impact of having HIV, ARC or AIDS on the respondents' sexual well-being. A range of factors can contribute to, or be symptoms of, depression which include a loss of sex drive and sexual dysfunction which may have an adverse impact on the individual's self-esteem and, in turn, on the lives of partners. Many voluntary and self-help organisations as well as statutory counselling services now recognise the importance of providing advice on sexuality and sexual expression within the context of safer sex practices.

This survey addressed the issue of sexual well-being from a service provision standpoint and did not enquire into the respondents' sexuality or sexual lifestyle. While approximately a third of respondents had sought specific help on sexual matters, there was a high level of awareness concerning safer sex and sexual transmission, with information being provided from a range of sources.

Many respondents had received some form of advice on sexual behaviour at the time of their antibody test although the quality of this advice varied and ranged from unhelpful proscriptive advice, for example, 'don't have sex', to more helpful counselling on how to adjust to living with the virus. Thirty two per cent of the sample stated that they had needed specific advice on their sexual well-being and had received it from a range of sources: voluntary groups, clinicians, other health service personnel and 'HIV counsellors' from statutory bodies.

The most frequently sought information concerned safer sex and the risks to self and to others (26 respondents). Twenty four respondents had required more comprehensive counselling to advise themselves or their partners on sexual matters, with a few respondents having experienced a period of celibacy following their diagnosis and 90 per cent having made some change in their sexual living. Respondents were asked whether they had made any conscious decision about becoming a parent in the future and 76 per cent said that they had made no decision or that the question was not applicable to them given their circumstances of sexuality. Of the 44 people who stated that they had made a conscious decision on this matter, the majority felt unable to have children in the future although seven respondents mentioned their desire to become either a natural or adoptive parent if this were possible. Three of the respondents stated that they had been sterilised since knowing that they had the virus.

2.3 Accommodation, Help in the Home and Transport

A number of questions were asked concerning accommodation, household amenities, the impact of HIV, ARC or AIDS on the accessibility and adequacy of housing and the requirement for specific amenities or household items.

Three-quarters of respondents lived in flats or rooms, with only 39 respondents (21 per cent) living in a house. Clearly there are a number of factors influencing accommodation type including cost, availability, and household circumstances. Table 2.21 shows the accommodation profile of the sample.

Table 2.21   **Type of Accommodation**

Type	Number	% Total
Flat (unspecified)	49	27
Flat (ground floor)	18	10
Flat (above ground floor)	59	33
Bedsit (unspecified)	7	4
House	39	21
Other including B&B hostel, rehab. unit and not known	9	5
Total	**181**	**100**

Where the location of the flat was unspecified, it may be assumed that a proportion of these will be on upper storeys as will a proportion of 'bedsits' and rooms in the 'other accommodation' category. On this basis, the number of people living in 'above ground' floor property is high and the figures of 34 per cent of people with ARC and 35 per cent of people with AIDS stating that they live above ground floor are undoubtedly underestimates.

Advice on Housing

Seventy three respondents (40 per cent of the sample) had sought advice or assistance concerning their housing:

- 51 people had sought help once
- 13 people had sought help twice
- 8 people had sought help three times
- 1 person had sought help four times.

However, the above figures do not take account of the overall contact that the respondents might have had with helping agencies whilst, for example, an application for housing was being pursued. Table 2.22 shows the sources of help.

Table 2.22 **Housing Problems: Sources of Help**

Source	No.
Local council	30
HIV-AIDS voluntary group	20
Social Services/Social Work dept	14
Hospital/HIV clinic staff (inc. hospital social worker)	13
Housing advice/welfare rights organis-ation	10
Housing association	8
Drugs group (voluntary and statutory)	4
Building society	2
Solicitor	2
Dept of Social Security	1

Alternative Accommodation

Public housing is the most frequently pursued option for alternative accommodation with less use made of housing associations, some of which now have considerable expertise in housing single people or people with mobility problems. Some concern was expressed that council housing might only be made available to people diagnosed with ARC or AIDS when people who were HIV positive might also face homelessness or have inadequate housing for their current or likely future needs.

When invited to give their recommendations on the type of housing and associated facilities which they felt should be provided for people with the virus, the following list in order of frequency emerged.

- Ground floor accommodation

- Internal and external adaptations to increase mobility

- Housing located close to services and amenities, eg clinics

- A wider choice of housing type and location to prevent 'ghettoisation'

- Cluster or sheltered housing where people with the virus can assist one another but with on-site support (and warden support in general)

- Housing to be located in quiet, 'low-risk' neighbourhoods

- The provision of equipment such as washing-machines etc which can be used by people with mobility/health problems

- A minimum of two-bedroom housing to accommodate carers

- Secure tenancies and rent agreements

- Furnished accommodation

- Adequate and affordable heating

- The installation of telephones and intercom systems for communication and personal security.

- Less 'bureaucracy' and increased confidentiality in respect of housing applications from people with the virus.

Forced Moves

Respondents were asked if they had ever had to move or leave home since having the virus and 51 respondents (28 per cent) stated that they had. The reasons for moving varied and these have been categorised as follows and shown in Table 2.23.

Harassment: reaction of others towards respondent because of HIV-AIDS, racism or homophobia

Property: housing inadequate or unsuitable for health needs

Drug use: problems with drug use or need for drug-related services

Relationships: personal relationships

Finance: financial problems/reasons to move

Care: desire/need for care or companionship

Other: for example, imprisonment, returning from abroad, burglary.

Table 2.23 **Reason for Moving Home**

Reason	Number[1]	Percentage of movers	Percentage of sample
Harassment	18	35	10
Property	11	22	6
Drug Use	6	12	3
Care	4	8	2
Other reasons	4	8	2
Relationships	3	6	1
Finance	3	6	1

[1] some respondents gave more than one reason for moving home.

The figures for 'harassment' given in Table 2.23 refer only to those situations which prompted the respondent to move home. When respondents were asked directly whether they had experienced any harassment or discrimination where they lived now or previously, 29 people (16 per cent of the sample) said that they had been discriminated against in some way. The figure for Scotland was highest with 26 per cent of respondents reporting incidents of discrimination. Harassment took the form of hostile reactions towards the respondents' sexuality, HIV status or culture, and showed itself in verbal abuse, eviction from public buildings or accommodation, threats or violence, graffiti on their homes, tradespeople refusing to carry out work and so forth.

Homelessness and Seeking Accommodation Change

Thirty three respondents (18 per cent of the sample) stated that they had been made homeless or had needed to rely on others to house them since knowing they had the virus. There were area variations in response to this question showing that 32 per cent Scottish respondents had been without their own accommodation; compared with 20 per cent of London respondents and 10 per cent of those in Manchester.

Almost a third of respondents (32 per cent) said that they were seeking a change of housing at the time they were interviewed with Table 2.24 shows that Scottish respondents were more dissatisfied with their current accommodation than those in the English cities.

Table 2.24 **Number of Respondents Seeking a Change of Housing**

Scotland (n=31)		Manchester (n=67)		London (n=81)	
No.	Percentage	No.	Percentage	No.	Percentage
17	55	21	31	20	25

The most frequent reason given for seeking a change of accommodation, stated by 45 per cent of those wishing to move, was that current housing was unsuitable either for current health needs or for longer-term health needs for example:

- a demand for ground floor accommodation because of mobility problems
- a demand for extra rooms to accommodate carers
- wanting a smaller more manageable property
- wanting to live in a better neighbourhood
- to be nearer to amenities and services

A desire for change because of 'personal' reasons was mentioned by 38 per cent of respondents wishing to move, for example:

- wanting to live independently
- wanting more secure tenure
- to make a 'fresh start'.

A desire for change centring on 'people', expressed by 21 per cent of those wishing to move, included:

- wanting to live with a partner or friends
- wanting to share with other people who were antibody positive
- wanting to move from unhappy relationships
- wanting to move from harassment/unfriendly neighbours

Stairs

To pursue the question of appropriate housing and accessibility further, respondents were asked whether the design or location of their housing caused them any problems. A total of 88 respondents (49 per cent of the sample) experienced some problems in using stairs (or steps) either in their own home, in other places, or both, and these included 83 per cent of those people with ARC and 72 per cent of those people with AIDS. It was interesting to note that 29 per cent of people who are HIV positive also had problems using stairs.

Those people having difficulty with stairs were asked whether or not they had access to a lift. Only 27 of the 88 respondents had access to a lift and 14 of these respondents stated that the lifts were frequently faulty. It is clear that respondents are concerned not only with their immediate requirements for accessible homes which maximise mobility but also with their future requirements should they fall ill. The comments received on housing also imply a strong belief in the association between stress/anxiety and deterioration of the immune system with a number of respondents referring particularly to the need for an appropriate and relaxing home environment.

The size of peoples' homes may be an important factor in ensuring that informal helpers and carers are able to be at hand if required. A total of 91 respondents (52 per cent of the sample) had no means of 'putting up' a friend or relative overnight, with respondents in Manchester less able to provide this facility (68 per cent of Manchester respondents).

The premium placed by respondents on independence, adequate space and the location of their homes is confirmed by the replies given to the question 'what are the good points about your housing?' where respondents listed a number of positive aspects of their current homes, the most frequent being:

- being near to amenities, shops and transport   — 54 (30 per cent of sample)

- living in a quiet, safe area   — 48 (28 per cent of sample)

- having freedom and independence   — 26 (14 per cent of sample)

- comfortable, well-equipped home   — 21 (12 per cent of sample)
- having a garden   — 19 (11 per cent of sample)
- having sufficient space   — 15 (8 per cent of sample)

Heating

A total of 84 people (48 per cent of the sample) said that they had problems in heating their homes and these problems have been categorised as shown in Table 2.25.

Table 2.25   **Heating Problems**

Problem	No	% of total sample n=181	% people with problems n=84	% Lon n=81	% Man n=48	% Scot n=31	% Birm n=19
Cost	57	31	68	27	21	42	58
Heating inadequate	44	24	52	28	21	13	32
Respondent person- ally cold	9	5	11	6	4	2	—
Continual faults	6	3	7	4	2	—	10

N.B. Some people gave more than one reason

Amenities and Household Items

Respondents were asked whether they had use of a number of household amenities and items. To try and assess the impact of HIV-AIDS on their daily needs, people were also asked whether their use of these items had changed since knowing they had the virus, and if so, in what way (Table 2.26).

The respondents were asked whether or not they had acquired any items for the home or domestic appliances since because of having the virus and 52 respondents (29 per cent of the sample) had acquired one or more such items. People with AIDS were most likely to have acquired items at 48 per cent, compared with 37 per cent of people with ARC and only 19 per cent of those who were HIV positive.

Table 2.26 **Use of Amenities Since Diagnosis**

	Bath	Shower	Toilet	Oven	Microwave	Fridge	Washing Machine	Phone
	%	%	%	%	%	%	%	%
Used More	25	19	26	10	30	17	34	47
Used Same	72	78	74	77	70	83	61	53
Used Less	3	3	—	13	—	—	5	—
n=	166	74	170	168	77	166	124	139

The most frequently acquired household item was a washing machine (17 respondents). Twelve respondents had acquired a microwave cooker and six respondents had installed a telephone. The categories of household items and appliances acquired are as follows:

Food preparation and cooking (27 respondents)
For example, food processor, cooker, microwave, refrigerator, freezer, blender

Housework (22 respondents)
For example, washing machine, vacuum cleaner, dishwasher, spin drier

Personal comfort/health (11 respondents)
For example, ioniser, humidifier, fan, heaters

Leisure/exercise (10 respondents)
For example, television, video, exercise equipment

Furniture (seven respondents)
For example, beds, bedding, furnishing house or flat throughout

Convenience (five respondents)
For example, jar openers, answerphone, intercom

The majority of the 97 items mentioned had been purchased or acquired by the respondents themselves or their families as shown in Table 2.27.

Approximately half of this sample (91 respondents) stated that they still required certain items for the home. The ten most frequently mentioned are listed below:

washing machine   (33 respondents)
microwave   (21)

41

clothes/spin drier	(15)
telephone	(15)
shower	(12)
refrigerator/freezer	(10)
vacuum cleaner	(6)
dishwasher	(6)
cooker	(4)
bed	(3)

Table 2.27   **Source of Funds for Purchase of Household Equipment**

Source	Number of Items
Self	53
Voluntary groups and charities	16
Social services/DSS	15
Family	7
NHS	2
Local council	2
Other	2

Practical Assistance in the Home

Respondents were asked to state whether they had ever needed practical assistance (as opposed to emotional support) with day-to-day activities and the questionnaire allowed for a maximum of eight separate activities per respondent to be reported. Because of the often fluctuating nature of illness associated with HIV infection and the fact that people may require assistance at different times, the respondents were asked to clarify whether or not help was currently required, or had been required in the past. In 38 cases the details of help required was unknown or the question had not been asked and therefore the findings of this section of the report may be an understatement of the actual demand for such support. A total of 84 respondents (46 per cent of the sample) stated that they had required assistance with one or more of a wide range of activities and this included four respondents whose single problem concerned transport. Discounting all transport problems which are discussed later in this chapter, the remaining 80 respondents (44 per cent of the sample) reported 230 problems (Table 2.28).

Table 2.28 **Practical Problems Reported by Respondents**

No. of Problems	No. of Respondents	Total Problems
1	22	22
2	21	42
3	11	33
4	10	40
5	7	35
6	6	36
7	2	14
8	1	8
Total	**80**	**230**

When the type of help required was categorised by the diagnosis of the respondent it was found that although those with ARC and AIDS required a wide range of help, people who were HIV positive only still required assistance with basic activities such as shopping and housework (Table 2.29).

Table 2.29 **Help Required with Activities by Diagnosis, Showing Percentage of Total Sample**

Help Required	HIV		ARC		AIDs	
	No.	%	No.	%	No.	%
Housework	16	15	15	43	23	58
Shopping	15	14	15	43	23	58
Laundry	16	15	8	23	15	38
Cooking	9	8	7	20	16	40
All Activities	30	28	22	63	28	70

Carers

Only a small number of people identified someone whom they defined as a 'carer'. Yet the information provided in this section of the survey confirms the respondents' widespread use of informal care, especially from friends and partners, to assist them with daily living activities. It may be that the respondents preferred not to define their friends or partners as 'carers' insofar as the term implies a relationship based on dependency; assistance with shopping or cooking, for example, may be seen as a reorganisation of responsibility for tasks rather than a formal acknowledgement of 'care' being received and given.

Only nine of the 181 respondents (5 per cent of the sample) was receiving the assistance of a Home Help at the time of this survey, with an additional three respondents due to have a Home Help in the near future.

When asked why a Home Help was not used, 142 respondents replied that they had 'no need' for this kind of support (Table 2.30). Only five of these respondents stated that this was because they had other people to help them.

Table 2.30   **Reasons for Not Having a Home Help**

Reason	Number of Respondents
No need	142
Application refused/cannot obtain	12
Don't know how to obtain	5
On waiting list	3
Does not want 'others' in his/her home	2
Help required spasmodically	2
Would feel guilty	1
Need only just arisen	1
(Not known)	4

Although a number of people required and received help with cooking and preparing meals, only five respondents (3 per cent of the sample) had received a meals service. All of them lived in London. At the time of this survey only three respondents were receiving meals, all from a voluntary organisation. Of the remaining 178 respondents, 154 stated that they had 'no need' for such a service.

Five respondents believed that they had been refused practical support in the home from another source because they had an informal helper: 'the social workers think you can cope', 'refused Home Help because of friend's help' and so forth.

Fifteen respondents had received advice concerning their mobility needs in the home and had received visits from the following statutory workers

- Occupational Therapist   — 7 respondents
- Home Support Team (or equivalent)   — 5
- Nurse/health advisor   — 4
- Community Psychiatric Nurse   — 1
- Voluntary Group Welfare Rights Officer   — 1

The fact that nearly half the sample required some form of assistance in the home but only 5 per cent of the respondents were receiving statutory assistance confirms the importance placed on informal care. There is a high demand for assistance yet a lower demand for the services currently provided by social service/social work departments and similar agencies which are often seen as being designed, available or appropriate for, people with severe disability or terminal illness.

Transport

Just over a quarter of the sample (28 per cent, 51 respondents) owned a car, 8 per cent (15 respondents) owned a bicycle, and a further 42 respondents (23 per cent) had access to a vehicle owned by a partner, friend or family member should they require a lift. This left approximately 40 per cent of people with the virus without a source of private transport.

The frequency of reported transport problems increased with the severity of the diagnosis, with 33 per cent of people HIV positive, 54 per cent of people with ARC, and 65 per cent of people with AIDS experiencing a transport problem.

The most common problem arose when respondents with mobility or health problems found transport inaccessible or travel in general too exhausting. This problem was cited by 61 respondents and included people who were too weak or fatigued to use public transport, those who needed mobility aids such as crutches or wheelchairs, and those who had extreme difficulty in walking. The second most common problem was with the availability of transport (33 respondents) who complained of infrequent or unreliable services and the distances required to travel to amenities. In addition, a total of

32 respondents mentioned their difficulty in affording transport and these included nine respondents who specifically cited their increased use of taxis. This problem was mentioned by a higher proportion of the Scottish respondents (78 per cent) than those from other areas. A further 11 respondents spoke of their difficulty in coping with city travel and here the problems of noise, traffic and the stress of using public transport were given as examples.

The respondents were asked which 'places' proved the most difficult to reach in terms of transport problems and the four most frequently mentioned places were:

- out-patient clinic/hospital   (25 per cent)
- shop/post offices/chemists (15 per cent)
- relatives   (14 per cent)
- leisure outlets/friends   (11 per cent)

The above figures should be seen in the context that a further 13 per cent of the respondents said that they had difficulty reaching 'everywhere' which can be assumed to include the above places.

A total of 62 respondents (34 per cent of the sample) said that they had changed their mode of transport to particular places as a result of having the virus. These respondents often reported more than one change of transport. The most frequent change was from the use of public transport to taxis (32 respondents) because of the inaccessibility of buses, the need for door-to-door facilities or due to the receipt of taxi cards (London). The main reason for taxi use was in relation to the problems posed by public transport for those with mobility or health problems.

Forty two respondents (24 per cent) had sought help with their transport problems from a variety of sources. The remaining 38 respondents had not sought help for a number of reasons including the following:

- 6 respondents said that they had 'managed' or had found solutions to their problems without formal assistance
- 6 did not know that help existed or who to contact
- 5 felt that they would not qualify for assistance
- 3 said that it had 'not occurred' to them to ask for help or advice.

People with ARC or AIDS were more likely to have sought assistance with transport, at 46 per cent and 40 per cent respectively, compared with 10 per cent of people who were HIV positive only.

The majority of respondents seeking help with transport problems approached more than one source of assistance (Table 2.31).

Table 2.31 **Transport Problems: Agencies Contacted (all respondents seeking help with transport problems)**

Social Services	31
Voluntary Groups	17
Dept of Social Security	12
Local Council	7
Consumer Organisation	1

The most frequent reason for seeking assistance from the above agencies was a requirement for help with the cost of transport either through the receipt of mobility allowance, or through an application for a taxi-card or other free or reduced fare concession (Table 2.32).

Table 2.32 **Transport Problems: Reason for Seeking Help[1]**

Taxi-card or similar	36
Mobility allowance	14
Financial assistance (general enquiry)	12
Disablement car sticker	3

[1] some respondents reported more than one reason for seeking assistance.

It was interesting to note that only one of the respondents originally seeking mobility allowance received it, although one other person was awaiting the outcome of a claim. The extent of formal assistance received with transport is demonstrated in table 2.33.

The provision of 'taxi-cards' was confined to London although railcards and travel passes of other kinds were available elsewhere.

Table 2.33   **Transport Problems: Formal Assistance**

Concessionary fare 'cards' or reimbursement of fares	34
On waiting list for financial help/'cards'	8
Help with lifts	8
Advice	4
Car badges	2
Received a car	1

When the respondents were asked whether they needed practical assistance in the home, 40 people chose to mention their need for assistance with transport (rather than transport costs) at this juncture and whilst this does not represent the total number of people who said that they experienced problems due to their mobility, levels of fatigue and so forth, the following findings show that whilst the use of informal care is high amongst this group, a majority of the 40 respondents did not have sufficient help with the practical aspects of transport (Table 2.34).

Table 2.34   **Level of Help from Various Sources**

Receives help from:	Number	Sufficient Help?		
		Yes	No	DK
No-one	13	—	13	—
Friend	10	6	3	1
Partner	5	4	1	—
Volunteer	5	3	2	—
Parent	3	1	2	—
Social Services	1	1	—	—
Nurse	1	1	—	—
Both informal and formal help	1	1	—	—
Not known	1	—	1	—
Total	**40**	**17**	**22**	**1**

The respondents were asked what changes they would like to see with regard to transport facilities and 105 respondents made one or more recommendations. A demand for improved public transport (and especially buses) was expressed by 63 respondents who mentioned the problems of bus-steps and overcrowding in particular. The question of financial assistance with fares, particularly taxi-fares, was raised by a number of respondents.

2.4 Paid Employment and Voluntary Work

Employment Status

The employment status of the 179 respondents who had left full-time education is shown in Table 2.35:

Table 2.35 **Employment Status**

	Number	% of total
Employed	69	39
Employed but on sickness leave	3	2
Unemployed—seeking work	26	14
Unemployed—not seeking work	64	35
Retired	17	9
Total	**179**	**100**

The data on people in employment refer to those 69 people at work at the time they were interviewed and exclude those people who were still employed but were on long-term sickness leave. A further 12 people were, in fact, away from work due to illness at the time they were interviewed but they did not classify themselves as being 'long-term sick'.

When these data were examined by HIV status it was found that 47 per cent of HIV positive respondents were working, 33 per cent of people with AIDS and 17 per cent of people with ARC.

Changes in Employment

The 69 respondents currently working were asked whether they had made any changes in their employment conditions since knowing that they had the virus and these changes are set out in the Table 2.36.

Table 2.36   **Employment Changes—Among Currently Employed**

Change	Number	Percentage
Changed job	16	23
Changed hours	13	19
Changed duties within same job	17	25
Changed location within same job	10	14

Of those 107 respondents who were not currently working, either because they had never had a job or had left employment, 51 (48 per cent) had worked at some time since having the virus. When the data on the year that respondents were last in paid employment were correlated with the year of their diagnosis (92 respondents) it was found that 38 per cent had left employment prior to diagnosis; 25 per cent had last had a paid job in the same year that they were diagnosed; and 37 per cent had left employment following diagnosis. Of those respondents leaving work following the year of diagnosis, 62 per cent had done so within the next two years.

Employment and Health

When respondents were asked whether they felt their working conditions had affected their health in any way, 77 people (63 per cent) felt that they had. The most frequent comment (42 people) was in relation to the problems of fatigue and stress at work, for example, the physical requirements of the job, the 'pace' of the working environment or the demand of working unsocial hours. A further 26 people spoke specifically about the emotional or psychological strain of working, particularly where colleagues did not know the individual's HIV status. Respondents mentioned, for example, the constant fear of people finding out, the need to explain frequent illnesses so as not to arouse suspicion, worries of contracting infections from co-workers or the rejection and hostility of others. Only six respondents mentioned the positive aspects of working and especially the fact that work 'kept them going'.

Employers' and Others' Knowledge of HIV Status

The experience of people in employment will, of course, be influenced by whether employers or colleagues know that the individual has the virus. The respondents were asked whether anyone at their place of work was aware of their HIV status, and if so, how they had been informed (Table 2.37).

50

Table 2.37   **Knowledge of Respondent's Status**

	Number	% of total (n=123)	% of those working (n=72)	% of ex-workers (n=51)
Status known	59	48	51	43
Status unknown	58	47	43	53
Don't know or not applicable	6	5	6	4
Total	**123**	**100**	**100**	**100**

A total of 10 respondents reported that 'everyone' they worked with knew of their HIV status; 22 respondents stated that their employer, 'boss' or 'superior' knew that the person had the virus, and 22 respondents stated that colleagues or certain friends at work were aware of their HIV status. In six instances the respondent's company or colleagues had been informed (or had found out) against the individual's wishes, for example through 'gossip', through other people informing the employer, through media publicity, or the respondent's admittance to a hospital ward identified with those who have the virus.

Respondents currently working and ex-workers (123 people) were asked whether they had experienced (or would expect) prejudice at work because of people's reactions to their HIV status. A total of 52 people (42 per cent) gave examples of their fears should their status be revealed:

Expectations

Different treatment: rejection, pampering, no understanding due to the ignorance of others.

Hostility: harassment.

Loss of work: would lose job, would be demoted, would lose custom/business, would lose money.

Experiences

Different treatment: rejection, avoidance, silence, over-protection; colleagues not sharing equipment.

Hostility: name-calling.

Loss of work: fired because of being HIV; fired because of sexuality.

Restrictions: not allowed to attend meetings; unable to join pension scheme; pension reduced but premiums not reduced.

Nevertheless, despite the fears and experiences of a number of respondents in this sample, 46 respondents gave examples of where colleagues or employers had been particularly supportive, by for example, re-arranging work schedules, allowing time-off, accepting the individual's condition, 'listening' and 'understanding'.

HIV and Employment Policy

The respondents working at the time they were interviewed were asked whether, to their knowledge, their employers had a specific policy regarding employees who had the virus. A total of 13 respondents out of 72 (18 per cent) said that they did not know or that such a policy was not applicable because, for example, the respondent was self-employed; 27 respondents (38 per cent) said that their employer did have some form of policy, either explicit or implicit concerning employees with the virus while 32 respondents (44 per cent) said that their employer did not have a policy. The policy most frequently mentioned was that of 'equal opportunities' or 'non-discrimination'.

Those respondents who had ceased work subsequently or who had not worked since knowing their HIV status (107 respondents) were asked whether they felt their unemployment or retirement had affected their physical or psychological health in any way. A total of 69 respondents (64 per cent) felt that their health had been affected, either positively or negatively, as a result of not working. When asked to classify in what way their health had been affected, these respondents reported as follows (some respondents gave more than one response):

[Feel] emotionally worse — 40 respondents (58%)
[Feel] physically worse — 5 respondents (7%)

[Feel] emotionally better — 11 respondents (16%)
[Feel] physically better — 16 respondents (23%)

A total of 173 people were asked if having the virus had changed their attitude towards work in any way and 59 per cent stated that their attitude had changed, resulting in either increased or decreased motivation to work. An examination of the comments received shows that over 80 of respondents whose attitude had changed had less motivation for work because of the problems they had encountered or feared that they would encounter. The responses to this question have been categorised and are shown below with examples (some respondents gave more than one reason for their change of motivation).

More Motivated

More career oriented: (13 replies)	want job more than ever; more determined; want to be successful; don't want the virus to interfere with work
Job improved: (7 replies)	more aware now of people's needs; work has improved; more assertive now; better at my job

Less Motivated

Changed priorities: (34 replies)	other things in life more important than work; career unimportant—just work for the money now; don't want to work—want to enjoy what life is left to me
Limitations on work: (25 replies)	could only work part-time due to fatigue; experience periodic illness; hospital appointments/check-ups would disrupt work; need to avoid stress; lack of concentration

Recommendations for Change

The respondents were asked for their recommendations in respect of support or services for people at work, or those wishing to work and 123 people gave their views which are shown in Table 2.38. The concern that is felt about discrimination in the workplace whether by colleagues, employers or customers and the influence such discrimination exerts on the ability or motivation to work is reflected in the number of respondents who responded to this question by stating that they wished to see wider 'education' of the factors surrounding HIV infection to dispel myths concerning transmission and to diminish the risk of rejection.

Table 2.38   **Recommendations for Support or Services for People at Work**

Recommendation	Number[1]
Increased education for the public	50
Increased education for employers	26
Increased education for employment agencies	16
Increased counselling/support	37
'HIV Policies' to prevent discrimination and dismissal or to support people	27

[1] Some respondents made more than one recommendation

53

A total of 39 people (22 per cent) had sought advice on workplace problems or on whether they should continue to work. The sources of advice were diverse and included job centres/agencies (the most frequently contacted), social workers, medical staff, voluntary groups, careers advisors, trade unions and so forth. Only five of these respondents stated that they had received no help following their enquiries, the majority of whom had contacted Job Centres.

The data collection in this survey on the health problems of people with the virus confirm that these problems should not be underestimated, but the number of people who, despite bouts of ill-health, remain fully active members of the community, suggests that with flexibility, imagination and an increase in awareness of the truth surrounding HIV infection, many more people with the virus could remain in work and gain an income sufficient for their needs.

Voluntary Work

'Voluntary organisations' refers to groups which may or may not be established for an HIV-specific purpose and which comprise volunteers who may or may not have the virus, for example, the Terrence Higgins Trust, Age Concern. The term 'self-help organisation' refers to those HIV-specific groups whose volunteers mainly comprise of people with the virus, for example, Body Positive, Positively Women. This sample of people with HIV, ARC or AIDS was recruited with the cooperation of a number of voluntary and self-help organisations and therefore the findings on participation in, or contact with, such organisations must be seen in that context. It was found that a third of this sample (33 per cent, 59 respondents) were active in one or more voluntary or self-help groups.

The respondents involved in voluntary work participated in a wide range of activities, the most frequently mentioned being:

- organisation and administration
- counselling and advice
- public speaking
- training
- telephone advice/helpline activity

Other work included buddying, fund-raising, practical help for people in their homes, writing articles and outreach work.

Table 2.39   **Participation in Voluntary or Self-Help Organisations**

Type of Organisation	No. of Respondents[1]	% Volunteers (n=59)
Self-help (eg Body Positive, Frontliners, Positively Women etc)	36	61
HIV-specific voluntary organisation (eg THT, local Aidsline, Act-Up)	29	49
Non HIV-specific voluntary organisation (eg youth group, Age Concern, church)	19	32
Drug-specific groups	6	10
Other	3	5

* respondents may belong to more than one group

The respondents were asked how many hours per week they spent on behalf of voluntary and self-help organisations. The average number of hours per week was 12, but this was within a range of between one or two hours per week to over 40 hours per week for some respondents. A total of 48 respondents (81 per cent of volunteers) said that they were more involved in voluntary work since having the virus.

The respondents were asked whether they felt any benefit from their voluntary activities and 55 respondents (93 per cent) said that they did. Those respondents involved in voluntary or self-help activity made a number of comments on the relevance that such activity had for their lives since having the virus and the most frequently expressed comment was the personal satisfaction and fulfilment gained from helping, giving or sharing with others. The second most frequent comment was that voluntary or self-help activity had provided a structure or focus for individual lives, for example, by providing a 'purpose' to life thus enabling respondents to live with their HIV status. Only two respondents mentioned some negative aspects of their voluntary work, for example feeling frustrated and angry or having difficulty giving public talks about their experiences.

2.5   Personal and Household Finance

The personal cost impact on an individual of living with HIV infection, ARC or AIDS is related to a number of personal circumstances:

- income and the effect of HIV status on earnings and on personal capital assets.

- employment situation and changes due to HIV status on the individual's use of time (for example, becoming a voluntary agency worker, etc).

- housing situation and the effect of HIV status on the adequacy of current accommodation.

- expenditure budget available for basic and non-essential items, and the effect of HIV status on this.

Variations in these circumstances between people with HIV infection, ARC and AIDS results in differences in personal cost impacts and the ensuing implications for employment, subsistence/maintenance and leisure.

Income

The respondents in the survey received income from two mains sets of sources: i. wages/salary and ii. benefits, occupational pensions, interest from shares/savings and other miscellaneous sources.

Seventy eight out of the 181 respondents received money from source i: on average £205 per week for those with HIV only, £113 for those with ARC and £198 for those with AIDS. One hundred and sixteen respondents received money from source ii: the sums were £62 for those who were HIV positive, £68 for those with ARC and £95 for those with AIDS. The total average weekly income for those in each diagnostic category was HIV positive £139, ARC £87 and AIDS £105.

In order to put these figures in context it is important to make an assessment of the impact on income of having the virus. The virus-related costs were identified in relation to lost income; additional home maintenance requirements, health maintenance; regular expenditure such as gas, telephone, insurance etc; and leisure and recreation. The impact of HIV-AIDS-related changes in expenditure on these items varied according to diagnostic category and are discussed below. A summary table of the various changes is presented at the end of the section (Table 2.49).

Assessment was made of the loss of earnings over the previous two years by respondents due to their having their virus. A weekly cost of lost earnings over this period was calculated for

i) respondents who were employed at the time of interview but had taken time off work because of their virus, and

ii) respondents who were not employed at the time of interview but had worked within the previous two years and had, whilst employed, taken time off because of the virus.

In addition, aggregate costs of lost earnings were estimated for the respondents who had become unemployed or retired prior to this two year period. Estimates of earnings lost were based on the average net weekly wage/salary of HIV positive, ARC and AIDS respondents (£205, £113 and £198 per week respectively). The personal cost impact of this can be examined for all respondents by their HIV status.

A total of 132 respondents had worked in the previous two years (78 per cent of all respondents not in full-time education). Of these, 33 respondents (25 per cent) are known to have incurred a loss of earnings from taking time off work over this time period due to having the virus (three cases unknown). The average is 38 weeks per person. Their earnings loss varied from a quarter of salary to respondents receiving no pay whilst off work. In total, over the two year period, losses amounted to an average cost of £67 per week for each of these respondents.

Table 2.40 demonstrates the higher element of earnings lost for each of the subsets of HIV positive, ARC and AIDS respondents who were not employed at the time of interview. However, the cost pattern is the same for the employed HIV positive, ARC and AIDS respondents. This high cost is related to the inclusion of the loss of earnings of those respondents who had been out of work for up to two years because of the virus. These included those taking early retirement and not seeking work at the time of the interview. Of the respondents not in full-time education, 37 (22 per cent) were long-term unemployed or retired (ie over two years). This group consisted of 13 people who were HIV positive (12 per cent), 14 with ARC (41 per cent) and 10 with AIDS (26 per cent). Table 2.41 shows the numbers of years since last employment for the long-term unemployed respondents. This was greatest for people with AIDS with an average of 5.6 years. This compared with about 4.5 years for HIV positive and 3.6 years for ARC respondents.

If it is assumed that all of this unemployment was related to having the virus, the total average cost of lost earnings up to interview time is estimated at £42,600 per person (at 1990 prices), or £47,500, £27,300 and

Table 2.40   **Earnings Loss over Previous Two Year Period**

Respondents who have worked in the past 2 years—weeks off work/earning loss	Diagnosis			
	HIV	ARC	AIDS	Total
Currently Employed				
No. of people	6	2	3	11
Average weeks out of work over the past 2 years	17	42	24	19
Average earnings loss (weekly) £'s over past 2 years	18	37	68	35
Currently Not Employed[1]				
No. of people	6	8	6	20
Average weeks out of work over past 2 years	24	35	78	48
Average earnings loss (weekly) £'s over past 2 years	54	60	150	85
All Respondents				
No. of people[2]	12	10	9	31
Average weeks out of work over past 2 years	19	43	60	38
Average earnings loss (weekly) £'s over past 2 years	36	55	123	67

[1] Not including respondents permanently retired (n=4)

[2] Not including two cases with unknown earning loss.

£57,700 for HIV positive, ARC and AIDS respondents respectively. Because some people were unemployed before they knew they had the virus, and others were out of work for other reasons, it is more realistic to assume less than 100 per cent lost earnings. If it is assumed that 50 per cent of the long-term unemployment of people who are HIV or have ARC and 75 per cent of that of people with AIDS is virus-related, then aggregate average costs of lost earnings up to the time of interview were £23,800, £13,600 and £43,200, for each HIV positive, ARC and AIDS respondent respectively.

Table 2.41 **Years Since Last Employment and Loss of Earnings**

Long Term Unemployed[1]	HIV	ARC	AIDS	Total
No. of people[2]	13	14	10	37
Average years since last employment	4.5	3.6	5.6	4.8
Average loss of earnings (total)				
High cost est. £000's[3]	47.5	27.3	57.7	42.6
Low cost est. £000's	23.8	13.6	43.2	25.2

[1] Excludes permanently retired (n=4)

[2] Excludes nine HIV+, two ARC respondents with unknown period of long-term unemployment.

[3] High cost estimate based on 100 per cent of long term unemployment years due to the virus, low cost estimate based on 50 per cent of HIV+/ARC unemployed years and 75 per cent of AIDS respondent unemployed years due to the virus.

Household Items

Table 2.42 shows that 52 respondents had obtained household equipment related to their having the virus. This represented 29 per cent of all respondents in the study. Items purchased included washing machines, cookers, sofa beds, telephones, stereos, videos, exercise equipment, ionisers and humidifiers. For these respondents, an average weekly cost of £1.25 per person for such equipment was estimated. This was based on an assumed seven year life of each item of equipment with the estimated actual cost as represented by its shop price discounted (at a 5 per cent rate to an average weekly cost over the life of the item). Discounting is a technique used to reflect the cost associated with future use of an item rather than focusing on an alternative use of the money spent on its purchase.

Six main areas of personal cost associated with the impact of HIV status on respondents' health maintenance were estimated. Changes were found in the personal costs of:

- diet/food
- health products from chemists/herbalists/health shops
- contraception and other sex products
- non-prescribed drug use
- smoking
- alcohol consumption

Table 2.42 **Weekly Cost of Household Equipment**

Source of expenditure on home equipment/appliances	HIV Status			
	HIV+	ARC	AIDS	Total
Respondent Expenditure[1]				
No. of people	14	9	11	34
Average personal cost (weekly) £'s	1.28	1.32	1.37	1.22
Statutory[2]				
No. of people	0	4	3	7
Average cost (weekly) £'s	—	0.99	0.47	0.76
Charity Expenditure[3]				
No. of people	7	5	4	16
Average cost (weekly) £'s	1.24	0.82	0.43	0.91
Total				
No. of People	20	13	19	52
Average cost (weekly) £'s	1.30	1.52	0.98	1.25

[1] Items purchased by the respondent or by his/her family

[2] DoH Health Authority, local authority

[3] Voluntary organisations, other charities

Food, Health Goods and Sex Products

Respondents were asked whether their expenditure requirements on food had changed because of having the virus. This was the case for 77 people (43 per cent of the sample) who said that they were facing higher food costs because of their condition. A total of 12 people (7 per cent of the respondents) said that food expenditure had decreased. Financial diaries completed over one week by 18 of the respondents, included details of expenditures on food prepared at home and that purchased outside (ie, cafes, restaurants, 'take-aways'). Table 2.43 shows that the average food-related expenditure for those respondents over one week was £49.72 per person, consisting of £27.09 and £22.63 per person on home prepared food and out-of-home meals respectively (the out-of-home figure includes some expenditure on alcohol where this formed part of the cost of meals).

Table 2.43   **Expenditure on Food**

Food/Meals	HIV	ARC	AIDS	Total
No. of people	9	2	7	18[1]
Average weekly expenditure home- prepared food £'s	21.98	24.48	34.41	27.09
out-of-home meals[2] £'s	21.32	40.24	19.29	22.63
Total weekly expenditure on food/ meals £'s	43.30	64.72	53.70	49.72

[1] One person with a home prepared food cost of £0.60 excluded

[2] Includes some alcohol expenditure (with meals)

However, because of the small number of people completing the diary and the fact that it was completed for one week only, the average food expenditure outcomes are only very tentative.

If the total average food expenditures drawn from the financial diaries are representative of the average for the whole sample then, as Table 2.44 shows for 43 per cent of respondents (ie those demonstrating an increase in food costs), it represents a higher cost than they would have incurred if they did not have the virus.

The purchase of health, herbal and alternative therapy produces represents a low cost method for improving psychological well-being in response to having the virus. In total 46 per cent of respondents (n=84) stated that because of having the virus they purchased additional health-related items such as vitamin tablets, aroma oils, garlic, disinfectant, royal jelly and relaxation tapes (see Table 2.44). There was only a small difference in the relative proportions of HIV positive, ARC and AIDS respondents who were purchasing health products because of the virus (see Table 2.49).

There was, however, a difference in the average weekly cost incurred by HIV positive, ARC and AIDS respondents on the purchase of health products. The lower average health product costs for people with AIDS and those who were HIV positive, were associated with the less frequent purchase of expensive products compared to the items obtained by respondents with ARC.

Only 13 per cent of the respondents (n=24) in the study had not made any changes to their sexual life since knowing they had the virus. The majority

Table 2.44   **Costs of Changes in Consumption of Food/Health Products**

Respondent food/health product cost	HIV Status			
	HIV	**ARC**	**AIDS**	**Total**
Food				
No. of people	12	6	5	23[1]
Average pre-virus cost (weekly) est.[2]				
£'s	33.33	52.51	39.59	39.69
Average current cost (weekly) est. £'s	41.17	60.70	51.71	48.56
Additional cost £'s	7.84	8.19	12.12	8.87
Health Products				
No. of people	43	15	14	72[3]
Average cost (weekly) £'s	2.56	4.91	3.26	3.18
Sexual Products				
No. of people	6	6	2	14
Average cost (weekly) £'s	2.94	2.66	0.92	2.53

[1] In total 42 people who were HIV positive had changed food expenditures (38 more cost, 6 less cost), 24 people with ARC had changed food expenditures (17 more, 7 less) and 23 people with AIDS had changed food expenditures (20 more, 3 less).

[2] Based on average food expenditures in the financial diary, with 10 per cent of the cost of meals out of home subtracted to account for any alcohol expenditures.

[3] Excluding seven people who were HIV positive, two people with ARC and three with AIDS for whom the cost of products purchased was unknown.

of these were people who were HIV positive (n=19). Only four people with AIDS (10 per cent of those making changes in their sexual life) incurred additional cost from the increased use of sexual aids. This represented an average cost of £0.92 per week incurred by two of the respondents for whom cost was known (see Table 2.44 above).

In contrast, 35 per cent of people with ARC who had made changes to their sexual life incurred greater personal cost as a result (n=11). This represented an increase in weekly personal cost of an average of £2.66 per person (for the six respondents for whom this cost could be quantified—Table 2.44). HIV positive respondents had incurred a cost through changes in their sex life associated with having the virus (at 21 per cent of all people who made some change, n=18), but at a greater weekly cost of £2.94 per person (for the six respondents for whom this cost could be quantified—see Table 2.44).

Illicit Drugs

Most of the drug using respondents were reluctant to divulge details of the expenditures they incurred through the purchase of non-prescribed drugs (eg heroin, 'speed', LSD). As Table 2.45 below shows, a total of 19 respondents stated that their use of drugs cost them money (10 people who were HIV positive, three with ARC and six with AIDS). This represented 54 per cent of all respondents who were using drugs (n=35). For people who were HIV positive, the range of weekly drug use expenditures (n=6) for those providing details was between £10 (two people) and up to £1,000 (one person). One person with ARC claimed weekly expenditures on drugs of £110. The respondents with AIDS provided estimates of personal cost of between £10 up to £2,100 per week (five people). Overall, the average weekly drug use expenditure for those providing information was over £300 per person.

Table 2.45   **Costs of Non-Prescribed Drugs**

	Non-prescribed drug use[1]	
HIV Status	**No. of People**	**Weekly Cost Range (£'s)**
HIV	10	10–1,000
ARC	3	110
AIDS	6	10–2,100

[1] eg Heroin, Cocaine, LSD, 'Speed', Amyl Nitrate

Tobacco

In terms of the distinction between HIV status, a greater proportion of people with AIDS had stopped or decreased their tobacco consumption relative to those who were HIV positive or who had ARC. Therefore, 30 per cent of pre-virus smokers with AIDS, compared to 17 per cent of pre-virus smokers with HIV positive/ARC respectively, obtained cost savings due to a reduction in tobacco consumption. However, the numbers of respondents providing details of changes in cigarette consumption were too small to accurately quantify the personal cost changes.

Alcohol

Table 2.46 demonstrates the high level of personal cost savings found for respondents from a net reduction in their average levels of alcohol consumption subsequent to diagnosis. A total of 132 respondents (73 per cent of the sample) stated that they were alcohol consumers prior to becoming HIV positive. Information on the weekly consumption of units of alcohol (one unit=half pint of beer, measure of spirits, glass of wine) both pre-virus and subsequent to acquiring the virus, was available for 109 respondents. In total, the average weekly pre-virus consumption was 29.5 units per person but was only 16.5 units at the time of the interview.

The net personal cost saving this represented was estimated to be £7.81 per person (based on a cost of £0.60 per unit of alcohol). This produced an average weekly cost of alcohol consumption of £9.91 per person, compared to £17.71 incurred by each drinker prior to becoming HIV positive.

Table 2.46   **Changes in Alcohol Consumption**

Alcohol Consumption since having the virus	HIV Status			
	HIV	**ARC**	**AIDS**	**Total**
Increased Consumption				
No. of people	8	5	0	13
No Change in Consumption				
No. of people	31	11	3	45
Decreased Consumption				
No. of people	25	9	17	51
Total No. of People	**64**	**25**	**20**	**109**
Average pre-virus weekly cost £'s	18.06	17.64	15.90	17.71
Average current weekly cost £'s	11.34	9.90	4.44	9.91
Net change in weekly cost £'s +/-	6.72	7.74	11.46	7.81

NB: Cost changes in consumption was unknown for 23 people consuming alcohol, who were excluded from the table.

Estimates based on numbers of units of alcohol consumed per week, estimate per unit cost of £0.60 eg the price of half a pint of lager).

Regular Household Expenditure

Table 2.47 outlines tentative findings regarding changes in three areas of regular household expenditures associated with respondents' HIV status.

Table 2.47   **Changes in Regular Household Expenses**

	HIV Status		
	HIV	**ARC**	**AIDS**
a) Change in Regular Expenditure			
No. of people with HIV related change	8	7	3
% of all respondents[1]	n/a	n/a	n/a
b) New Bills Since Virus			
No. of people[2]	16	15	25
% of respondents	(15)	(42)	(63)
c) Insurance Purchased Since Virus			
No. of people	4	2	3
% of respondents with insurance	(11)	(22)	(25)
Personal Cost[3]			
Average regular exp. pre-virus (weekly) £'s (all respondents)	14.50	13.49	17.35
Average regular exp. current (weekly) £'s	17.80	18.89	22.30
Change in personal cost (weekly) £'s +/- (all respondents)	+3.30	+5.40	+4.95

[1] The actual number of respondents with an HIV related change in regular expenditures is currently being determined. The numbers in the table are an underestimate, based on current numbers known to have experienced a change in regular expenditures due to HIV status.

[2] Of these six people HIV+, five people with ARC, one person with AIDS provided information on costs.

[3] Composite cost estimate based on a/b/c changes above.

The areas far which expenditures were assessed are as follows:

1. Regular expenses that had been experienced prior to acquiring the virus (eg electricity/gas, telephone, general living costs)

2. New expenses incurred since acquiring the virus (eg solicitor, hire purchase, transport)

3. Purchase of new insurance schemes (eg life insurance, hospital plans, plus contents insurance).

Assessment of changes because of the virus proved difficult, due to a high level of uncertainty amongst respondents regarding the extent to which any changes were due to HIV status.

Leisure and Social Interests

Having the virus had a significant impact on respondents' expenditures on leisure and social interests. Respondents were asked to estimate changes in expenditure on two sets of activities:

- Activities undertaken prior to acquiring the virus

- New activities taken up subsequent to acquiring the virus.

A total of 81 respondents provided information on their expenditures on a range of activities prior to acquiring the virus and subsequent changes. Data covered sport and recreation interests, hobbies, social events and other non-work, non-basic subsistence activities (drug use expenditures were, however, excluded).

As Table 2.48 shows, having the virus resulted in a large reduction in average expenditures on leisure/social interests.

From an average pre-virus weekly expenditure on leisure/social interests of £51.90, the respondents with AIDS demonstrated, on average, a decline in expenditure of £44.43 per person (n=21). A total of 43 per cent of respondents with AIDS incurred expenditures on activities taken up since becoming HIV positive. The average weekly cost for this group was found to be £5.69 per person. On this evidence, the net personal cost impact estimated for all AIDS respondents was a reduction in weekly expenditures of £41.98 per person (to £9.92).

Table 2.48   **Changes in Costs of Leisure and Social Interests**

Leisure/Social Interests	HIV Status		
	HIV	ARC	AIDS
Pre-virus activities			
No. of people[1]	43	17	21
Average pre-virus cost (weekly) £'s	24.33	47.72	51.90
Average current cost (weekly) £'s	14.69	14.38	7.47
Change in cost +/- (weekly) £'s	−9.64	−33.48	−44.43
New activities			
No. of people	43	19	17
% of respondents	(41)	(54)	(43)
Average current cost (weekly) £'s	8.30	2.88	5.69
All activities			
Average current cost est. (weekly) £'s	18.09	15.94	9.92
Net change in cost (weekly) +/− £'s	−6.24	−31.78	−41.98

[1] This was the number of respondents providing details of pre-virus cost and leisure interests and change in cost after acquiring the virus. In total, n=157 provided details of pre-virus leisure activities undertaken.

There is a need for these cost impact comparisons to be treated with some caution. Firstly, in determining the net change in leisure/social interest expenditures for all respondents, it has been assumed that the average expenditures for the 81 respondents who provided details on change costs, were representative of the whole study sample (n=181). Secondly, the pre-virus weekly average expenditures on leisure/social pursuits estimated for respondents who were HIV positive was much lower (at £24.33 per person) than that of the other respondents. The retrospective assessment of pre-virus costs may have resulted in some degree of overestimation of these expenditures by people with ARC/AIDS and/or some underestimation of cost by people who were HIV positive. If so, this may have been due to the greater magnitude of change in personal social/leisure activity recorded for the former group.

Summary of Financial Impact

Data presented in this section are summarised below in Table 2.49:

Table 2.49   **Personal Financial Impact of Living with HIV-AIDS**

Average Change in Personal Cost per Individual Experiencing a Change Since HIV Diagnosis		HIV+ (n=106)	ARC (n=35)	AIDS (n=40)
Average earnings per week		£205	£113	£198
Earnings loss per week[1] (over past 2 years)		£36	£55	£123
% of respondents		11	29	23
Long term unemployment[1] (ie exceeding 2 years)				
Loss of earnings since	High	£47,500	£27,300	£57,700
diagnosis[2]	Low	£23,800	£13,600	£43,200
% of respondents affected		12	41	26
Household equipment cost per week		+£1.28	+£1.32	+£1.37
% of respondents		13	26	28
Changes in Food cost per week[3]		+£7.84	+£8.19	+£12.12
Health products cost per week		+£2.56	+£4.91	+£3.26
% of respondents		40	43	29
Sexual products cost per week		+£2.94	+£2.66	+£0.92
% of respondents		5	17	5
Alcohol cost per week		–£6.72	–£7.74	–£11.46
% of respondents		60	71	50
Regular household bills—cost per week[3]		+£3.30	+£5.40	+£4.95
Leisure/social costs per week[3]		–£6.24	–£31.78	–£41.98

Notes

A negative sign demonstrates a reduction in expenditure, a positive sign an increase in expenditure (1989 prices) for respondents experiencing a change in costs incurred since having the virus.

[1] Not including income from benefits/other sources.

[2] High estimate based on the assumption that 100 per cent of long-term unemployment was due to the virus; low estimate based on 50 per cent of HIV+/ARC, and 75 per cent of AIDS, long-term unemployment was due to the virus.

[3] Covers average change in costs for all respondents in the sample.

3 Using Informal and Formal Social Care

3.1 Use of Antibody Testing Services

All of the respondents in the sample had their HIV status confirmed by antibody testing. Since living with HIV-AIDS has an enormous impact on an individual's daily life, it is important to recognise the immense psychological impact of being diagnosed in the first place.

The majority of respondents in the sample (83 per cent) were antibody tested at their nearest (local) hospital with few respondents using private testing facilities or general practitioners. Just three respondents chose to be tested at hospitals in other towns because of their concerns with confidentiality (Table 3.1).

Table 3.1   **Antibody Testing Site (n=181)**

Site	No.	Percentage of Sample
Local hospital	151	83
GP	9	5
Non-local hospital	3	2
Private test site	2	1
Other	14	8
Not known	2	1
	181	100

NB 'Other' includes detoxification centres, antenatal clinics, haemo-
philia centres, blood transfusion services and 'abroad'.

The majority of respondents (139) had chosen the test site thenselves because they were either familiar with the clinic (for example, a genito-urinary medicine department or a sexually-transmitted diseases clinic) or were aware that it was the local testing site. Only five respondents mentioned specifically being referred to the test site by a general practitioner. A total of 15 respondents had the HIV antibody test whilst they were hospital inpatients.

The majority of people in the survey (80 per cent) had requested or agreed to have antibody testing (Table 3.2). However 14 per cent were tested without their consent or knowledge and 3 per cent found they were HIV positive following a routine test, for example via blood donation. None of the Birmingham respondents were tested without giving consent, although two people from Birmingham had received results following blood donations. However 21 per cent of Manchester respondents, 15 per cent of London respondents and 13 per cent of Scottish respondents were tested without their knowledge.

Table 3.2 **Circumstances of the Antibody Test (n=181)**

	No.	Percentage of Sample
Requested/agreed to test	145	80
Tested without consent/knowledge	26	14
Routine test eg, via blood donation	5	3
Asked to participate in survey	2	1
Not known	3	2
	181	100

The number of people not giving informed consent for testing is small and an examination of these data by the year of diagnosis suggests a decrease over time in the proportion of people being tested without their consent.

The respondents who had sought testing discussed their personal reasons for seeking an antibody test. The most frequent reason for being tested can be classified as either a specific or a general suspicion that one might have the virus, for example, because of current or past sexual or drug-using activity, because of having received Factor 8, or because of a partner's HIV positive status. A total of 93 respondents (60 per cent of those who were aware of being tested) mentioned this reason. An alternative or additional reason for seeking testing was the experience of ill-health which was mentioned by 74 respondents or 48 per cent of those people who were aware of being tested. A total of 14 respondents (9 per cent of those seeking testing) stated that they had been tested in the firm belief that this would confirm they did not have the virus.

Counselling

Despite the fact that the majority of people in this sample had sought a test or agreed to a test being carried out, a high percentage of the total sample

(61 per cent) had no counselling prior to being tested. No pre-test counselling was given to 47 per cent of those people who had asked to take the antibody test.

The figures shown in Table 2.2 above suggested that the availability of pre-test counselling has increased over time, with 67 per cent of those tested in 1989 receiving pre-test compared with 23 per cent in 1984. The drug users in this sample were less likely to have received pre-test counselling: only 30 per cent of drug users receiving pre-test counselling, against 41 per cent of non drug users.

The people who had not received pre-test counselling were asked whether they would have liked this form of advice. A total of 67 out of 111 people (61 per cent) said that they would have liked information and advice prior to being tested. A further eight respondents (7 per cent) said they were not sure and in two cases preferences are unknown. It is interesting to note, however, that 34 respondents (31 per cent of those not counselled) stated that they would not have liked pre-test counselling, the most frequently expressed reason being an assumption that a counsellor would have tried to dissuade the individual from being tested.

A majority of the 70 people who had been counselled (39 respondents, 56 per cent) had been seen by someone they described as a 'health advisor' or 'HIV counsellor'. A further three respondents (4 per cent) stated specifically that they had been counselled by a social worker. It is not always possible for respondents to identify the precise professional title or role of the person counselling them and therefore a proportion of those staff referred to as 'counsellor' may, in fact, be hospital social workers, nurses or other professionals. A total of 22 respondents (31 per cent) had been given advice by a 'hospital doctor' or consultant and two people (3 per cent of those counselled) had been given advice by a general practitioner.

The attitude of the counsellor towards the individual being tested was considered to be in favour of testing in 36 per cent of cases, against testing in seven per cent of instances and neutral in 49 per cent of cases. In six cases the counsellor's attitudes was not known. There were some regional variations in respondents' opinions on this point. In London, 11 per cent of those counselled felt that the counsellor was in favour of testing compared with 56 per cent in Manchester and 58 per cent in Scotland. Similarly, 64 per cent of the London respondents felt that their counsellor showed a 'neutral' attitude, compared with 39 per cent in Manchester and 25 per cent in Scotland.

Whilst there still remains the question of informed consent in the testing of blood, it might be argued that in certain situations, clinicians or others may require to know quickly whether an individual carried the virus in order, for example, to provide appropriate treatment rapidly and that therfore there will be occasions when thorough counselling prior to a diagnosis is not possible. Where blood is taken via the blood transfusion service it is recognised that there is little opportunity to provide a counselling service prior to testing. However, there can be few situations where it is not poss-ible to provide counselling and advice once an antibody test result is known. It was therefore interesting to find that 69 people in this sample (38 per cent) received no counselling or advice following their diagnosis.

It was found that 35 per cent of those people seeking a test received no post-test counselling. In addition half of the respondents who had been tested without their knowledge received no post-test counselling and there-fore had received no form of advice either before or immediately following their diagnosis.

Out of the total sample, 63 per cent of non-drug users and 55 per cent of drug users had received post-test counselling. A total of 49 out of the 69 people who had not had any post-test counselling (71 per cent) stated that they would have liked to receive this form of advice. In nine cases the respondents' preference was not known. A further 11 respondents (16 per cent) stated that they did not want or need this kind of advice, for example, because they were already well informed (three respondents participating in HIV-AIDS voluntary organisations) or they had found the testing experience and the news of their diagnosis too traumatic and did not wish to prolong the experience (eight respondents).

When the respondents who had received post-test counselling were asked who had provided this service, the majority of respondents (61 per cent) had seen a 'counsellor' or 'health advisor' and 11 of these 68 respondents mentioned specifically that they had spoken to a hospital social worker. A further 38 respondents (34 per cent) had spoken to a medical professional, for example, a consultant, 'hospital doctor' or a nurse and three respon-dents also saw either a psychiatrist or a psychologist at the time of their diagnosis. Only three respondents had been given their post-test infor-mation by a member of an HIV-AIDS voluntary organisation.

There are many counselling methods and practice may differ between test-ing sites and the respondents were not, therefore, expected to assess or describe the counselling techniques used. However, the respondents were invited to comment on whether or not they had found the post-test counselling helpful. In general post-test counselling was considered to be helpful by two-thirds of respondents but there were significant regional variations. In Manchester and Birmingham post-test counselling was found to be helpful by 75 per cent and 83 per cent of respondents respectively compared with 57 per cent for London and 53 per cent in Scotland.

It is expected that people will find antibody testing a traumatic and distressing experience. Indeed, when asked whether they had any general comments to make, only 23 of the 109 respondents wished to record that they had experienced 'no problems' during the testing procedures or that the counselling and advice had been 'very good'. The comments made by the remaining 86 respondents revealed a number of very poor experiences, particularly relating to staff attitudes and statements made by members of staff to the respondents. A number of respondents gave graphic personal accounts of such negative reaction which are best categorised as follows:

i)   Problems with counselling

These respondents reported their dissatisfaction with either not receiving any counselling, or receiving poor quality advice, for example, a lack of 'practical' advice; inappropriate advice for women; 'misinformation' eg, HIV=death; proscriptive advice eg, 'never to have sex'; hostile attitudes.

ii)   Personal distress

These respondents' experiences were influenced by their personal reaction to a positive diagnosis, for example, shock and disbelief, or their distress at waiting for the test results. Other respondents mentioned their problems in coping with 'follow-up' medical procedures or the fact that they had not been tested because of subsequent problems in coping with the knowledge of their diagnosis.

iii)   Lack of follow-up

These respondents felt that there was insufficient 'follow-up' to check on their circumstances and would have liked a second-stage of counselling. Additionally they felt the test site staff to be too 'casual' or 'uncaring' with regard to their individual needs.

Confidentiality

A few respondents reported that their test result has been divulged to others, for example, employers and the media.

In addition to the above comments, a further 13 respondents felt that whilst their experience of antibody testing and counselling had been poor this was not due to any particular failure of procedures or a hostile reaction, but was almost inevitable given the level of knowledge concerning HIV-AIDS at the time they were tested. These respondents often remarked that they believed counselling and testing had improved greatly since their own experience. These comments reflect the findings of this survey when the data on 'good' and 'bad' experiences of testing are analysed by the respondents' year of diagnosis. These data show a decline in the proportion of people reporting 'bad' experiences since 1986—from 86 per cent in that year to 29 per cent in 1989.

The findings of this survey and the qualitative information provided by the respondents during interview confirm the important role played by effective pre- and post-test counselling. The impact of learning that one has the virus cannot be understated and the responsibility placed on counsellors to mitigate this impact and promote access to a range of support services is great. Those respondents who had not received counselling, or who had been dissatisfied with the nature or quality of the advice given had experienced immediate distress, anger or frustration and had, from their personal accounts, felt less equipped subsequently to cope with their diagnosis. The findings of the survey suggest that the availability and quality of counselling at testing sites has improved over time as awareness of the issues surrounding HIV-AIDS and the expertise of staff has developed. Nevertheless, this sample of people with HIV, ARC or AIDS contained a substantial number of people who were diagnosed within the last two years without counselling support. The number of respondents in this sample who were antibody tested without their knowledge or consent is also worth noting particularly in regard to the practice of testing for HIV antibodies during 'screening' for cause of illness. The low involvement of general practitioners in antibody testing and counselling is confirmed by this study.

For some of the people interviewed in this survey, the antibody test served to confirm what they suspected was their HIV positive status, but for others the diagnosis was a traumatic shock. To mitigate any adverse psychological reaction to a positive diagnosis and permit the individual to gain control over his or her life, it is necessary to ensure that pre-test counselling is sufficiently thorough to prepare the individual for the outcome of the antibody test. A negative test outcome may also have implications for future activity.

However, even where pre-test counselling has been undertaken, and whatever the individual's personal prediction of the test outcome might be, the news of seropositivity may invoke a range of reactions including initial disbelief or denial, anger or panic, and acute anxiety, perhaps to the extent of suicidal intent. An outwardly calm acceptance of the news may, in itself, be a form of denial. In a pre- or post-test counselling context, there is a clear need for staff at testing sites to ensure that each individual has the necessary information, advice and support with which to cope (a) in the immediate aftermath of the diagnosis and (b) in the longer term.

An antibody testing site will, in the majority of instances, be the first point of contact between the HIV positive individual and statutory sector services. As such the onus is on the test site counsellors to ensure that the individual is provided with information on how to gain access to health and social services should they be required in the future. Similarly, information concerning appropriate self-help and voluntary organisations should be made available. The majority of respondents in this sample were antibody tested in the last five years and it is important to emphasise that in Britain, as elsewhere, testing and counselling procedures have developed over time in terms of the availability of testing sites, the procedures adopted, and the training and expertise of test site staff.

3.2 Informal Care

This section examines the extent to which respondents rely on friends, partners and family—'informal carers'—for both practical assistance with day-to-day tasks and activities and for emotional support.

Practical Assistance

Half of the sample (88 respondents, 49 per cent) stated that someone regularly helps them or has done so in the past. There is some variation by diagnosis, with 68 per cent of respondents with AIDS reporting someone regularly helping, compared with 54 per cent of respondents with ARC and 40 per cent with HIV. Respondents in Scotland rely/relied more heavily on informal carers, with 77 per cent reporting that someone regularly helps, compared with 46 per cent in London, 48 per cent in Manchester and only

21 per cent in Birmingham. The relatively low figure for Birmingham can in part be explained by the fact that 74 per cent of respondents were HIV+. Table 3.3 shows the relative importance of different sources of informal care as used by respondent:

Table 3.3   **Informal Care—Persons Reported to be Regularly Helping Respondents (as a per cent of those specifying informal carers)**

Carer	HIV		ARC		AIDS		Total	
	No.	(%)	No.	(%)	No.	(%)	No.	(%)
Friends	30	(71.4)	14	(73.7)	10	(37.0)	54	(61.4)
Family	7	(16.7)	6	(31.6)	12	(44.4)	25	(28.4)
Partners	13	(31.0)	8	(42.1)	11	(40.7)	32	(36.4)
Neighbour/ flat mate	3	(7.1)	—	(—)	3	(11.1)	6	(6.8)
Other[1]	2	(4.8)	3	(15.8)	4	(14.8)	9	(10.2)
Total	42		19		27		88	

[1] includes: voluntary organisations, self-help groups and hospital counsellors.

There is considerable variation in terms of diagnosis when looking at the people who support/have supported respondents. People with HIV are more likely to receive support from friends (71 per cent, n=30) than are people with AIDS (37 per cent, n=10). Conversely respondents with AIDS cited family as carers in 44 per cent of cases (n=12), compared with only 17 per cent of respondents with HIV (n=7). The figures reflect those in Chapter 2 which suggest that respondents were more likely to tell friends of their HIV status than their families. As well as friends and family, a considerable proportion or respondents mentioned partners as sources of informal care and support (36 per cent, n=32).

Emotional Support

The majority of the sample looked to their family and friends for emotional support, with 83 per cent (n=150) reporting that they were able to talk over worries and problems with friends, relatives and partners. This emotional support was particularly important for respondents with AIDS (93 per cent, n=37), compared with 80 per cent of respondents with ARC and HIV (n=28

Table 3.4   **Informal Care: Sources of Emotional Support (as a percentage of respondents specifying sources of emotional support)**

Carer	HIV		ARC		AIDS		Total	
	No.	(%)	No.	(%)	No.	(%)	No.	(%)
Friends	30	(46.2)	12	(52.2)	17	(58.6)	59	(50.4)
Family	24	(36.9)	4	(17.4)	9	(31.0)	37	(31.6)
Partner	21	(32.3)	7	(30.4)	8	(27.6)	36	(30.8)
Other[1]	2	(3.1)	2	(8.7)	1	(3.5)	5	(4.3)
Total	**65**		**23**		**29**		**117**	

[1] includes: voluntary organisations, self-help groups and hospital counsellors.

NB: Some respondents named more than one person.

and 85 respectively). Table 3.4 shows the relative importance of different informal carers as sources of emotional support.

Compared with informal care in general, variations in the sources of emotional support between respondents with HIV, ARC and AIDS are less distinct. For example, friends were reported to give emotional support by 50 per cent of respondents, and this figure was only slightly higher for respondents with AIDS (59 per cent) than for those with HIV (46 per cent).

These figures contrast with those for informal care in general which show 71 per cent of respondents with HIV relying on friends, 73 per cent of those with ARC and only 37 per cent of those with AIDS.

Help for Carers

Some respondents (14 per cent of the sample, n=26) reported that a carer had sought practical help or advice because the respondent had the virus. There is some variation by diagnosis, with 25 per cent of carers of respondents with AIDS seeking help, compared with only 9 per cent of those respondents with HIV.

In the majority of cases (n=18), carers sought either HIV information or counselling. In ten cases informal carers received advice or help from voluntary organisations (39 per cent of those seeking help), in nine cases from a medical agency (35 per cent) and in only one case from a member of social services (4 per cent).

3.3 Use of the Voluntary and Self-Help Sector

Chapter 2 discussed the level of participation in voluntary work by people with HIV, ARC or AIDS. This section discusses the use made of voluntary or self-help groups and the same definitions of these groups apply, namely:

self-help — for example, Body Positive, Frontliners, Positively Women, Mainliners etc.

HIV-specific — for example, Terrence Higgins Trust, Scottish AIDS Monitor, local HIV/AIDS support group etc.

non HIV-specific — for example, gay/lesbian switchboard, church groups, legal/income/housing rights organisations etc.

In addition to the above three categories, there are groups established to advise or support drug users which, whilst not being HIV-specific, may offer particular services for ex or current drug users with the virus.

Level of Service Use

A large majority of the sample had made use of non-statutory groups in respect of services relating to their HIV status. Table 3.5 shows the numbers of respondents who had used voluntary or self-help organisations, by area.

Table 3.5 **Use of Voluntary or Self-Help Organisation by Area**

Area	No.	%
London (n=18)	60	74
Manchester (n=48)	34	71
Scotland (n=31)	30	97
Birmingham (n=19)	11	58
Total (n=181)	136[1]	75

[1] These figures include 1 from pilot study.

The lower figure for Birmingham may be accounted for by the fact that there are a higher proportion of HIV positive respondents from that area, since people with ARC or AIDS are more likely to have used a voluntary sector organisation (91 per cent and 78 per cent respectively) than are people who are HIV positive (69 per cent).

Most of the people included in the study (52 per cent) had used more than one voluntary or self-help group, although there were regional variations due mainly to the local availability of services. Respondents in London had a wider range of non-statutory services available to them, including multi-purpose centres such as the London Lighthouse and the Landmark Centre, and the large majority of those living in London (73 per cent) had used more than one voluntary or self-help group.

In order to ensure that users receive the most effective help and support available, it is important that they are well informed about the variety of voluntary and self-help groups and the services which they provide. Respondents reported that they found out about groups and services from a variety of sources. In just over a third of cases, respondents had been 'referred' to the voluntary group or advised of its availability by a member of hospital or social services staff, for example a hospital social worker. Other sources of information included the media and publicity material, voluntary sector referral and family or friends. In London, people were less likely to be referred to voluntary groups by the statutory sector, but were far more likely to have heard about voluntary or self-help groups through the media, posters and publicity leaflets. Only two respondents from Scotland (n=48) and none from Birmingham (n=12) reported that they had used media or publicity information.

Type of Service Use

The following Table 3.6 shows that the respondents in this sample most frequently used a self-help group (45 per cent). Since self-help groups such as Body Positive and Frontliners were foremost in assisting this project by publicising the survey, the pattern of self-help should be seen in this context.

A different pattern of voluntary group use was found for the drug users in the sample, where the most frequently used type of group was an HIV specific voluntary organisation (50 per cent). Self-help bodies accounted for 24 per cent of this group's use of voluntary services and specific drug related services represented 15 per cent.

Table 3.6   **Type of Voluntary or Self-Help
Organisation Used (n=263)**

	No.	%
Self-Help	117	45
HIV-specific	114	43
Non-HIV	15	6
Drug user group	11	4
Not known	6	2

Reasons for Use of Self-Help and Voluntary Organisations

People used self-help and voluntary organisations for a variety of purposes ranging from one-off requests for financial assistance to long-term use of a group for emotional support or social contact. Table 3.7 gives the frequency of reasons why people used these groups and shows the importance placed on peer-group support, emotional help and, 'understanding'. The use of voluntary groups for practical help appears to be more limited, although the figures may under-estimate the importance of informal networks of support gained via these organisations, for example where assistance at home results from friendships made through the organisation.

Although the users of drug agencies are slightly less likely to look for peer-group support or counselling from the agency than are users of other types of voluntary and self-help organisations, they are far more likely to use the group for 'social' reasons. During interview, current drug users frequently mentioned that the particular drug support group was their only social contact and was used as a focal point for meeting other drug users. In contrast some ex-drug users specifically mentioned that they were deterred from using drug related agencies because of their need to distance themselves from current users and remain abstinent.

In addition to the reasons given for using the voluntary and self-help organisations, it becomes apparent that some respondents received unlooked-for benefits from their use of the group. Whilst only two per cent of people gave 'Practical help in the home' as their reason for using a voluntary or self-help organisation, in fact eight per cent mentioned that they had received practical help such as cleaning and decorating and a further eight per cent had a 'buddy' to provide befriending support and/or practical

Table 3.7   **Reasons for Using Voluntary or Self-Help Organisations (by type of organisation)**

	Total %	Self-Help %	HIV %	Non HIV %	Drug %
Peer-group support and 'understanding'/ counselling	36	39	34	43	29
Legal and financial assistance	21	19	23	25	13
Health-related advice/health maintenance	10	11	10	1	—
Social contact/leisure	7	7	6	5	24
Housing	6	6	7	9	5
General advice/information	5	7	5	5	5
Transport	4	2	4	6	2
Safer sex advice/condoms	3	3	2	3	2
Practical help in the home	2	1	3	3	—
Drugs advice/needle exchange	2	1	2	—	20
Holidays	2	2	3	—	—
Help for carers	1	1	0.5	—	—
Antibody testing	1	1	0.5	—	—

help. Similarly, although only 10 per cent of respondents referred to the use of voluntary organisations for health manin/tenance therapies or 'treatments', 18 per cent of the total sample had participated in one or more health maintenance therapies via the voluntary sector.

When these data were examined in relation to respondents' HIV status a number of differences emerged between those who were HIV positive, had ARC or AIDS. Overall, these differences reflected the increased needs for practical support of those with illness and the worsened economic circumstances of those people unable to work compared with people who were HIV positive:

- Twice as many people with ARC or AIDS required legal and financial assistance;

- Twice as many people with ARC or AIDS required help with transport;

- Three times as many people with ARC or AIDS required help in the home and holidays.

The respondents were asked which was the most helpful activity or service provided by voluntary organisations and the most frequently cited activity (34 per cent) was peer group support. This was most often expressed as the need not to 'feel alone' with respondents deriving considerable reassurance from the support and empathy of others in a similar situation to themselves. In an additional 31 per cent of cases, the respondents said that overall emotional support and counselling (not necessarily provided by others with the virus) was the most helpful service provided (Table 3.8).

Table 3.8 **Most Helpful Services Provided by Voluntary or Self-Help Organisations**

Service	%
Peer group support	34
Emotional support/counselling	31
General advice and information	13
Benefits, advice and financial help	9
Practical help in the home	4
Drug-related advice and help	2
Housing	1
Anti-stress	1
Other	5

Quality of Service

In general the quality of the services provided by the voluntary and self-help organisations was considered to be good. The majority of respondents (54 per cent of 73 respondents) were of the opinion that, overall, voluntary services were 'excellent', 'very useful' or 'good'.

However, there were some reservations about different aspects of the voluntary services, and 53 per cent of those responding to the question (n=137) mentioned one or more problems that they had experienced or concerns that they had about the organisation or provision of voluntary support. People with ARC or AIDS reported dissatisfaction more frequently than those who were HIV positive (60 per cent and 46 per cent respectively). More Scottish respondents reported dissatisfaction (83 per cent) compared with respondents from London (63 per cent), Manchester (26 per cent) and the respondents from Birmingham, none of whom reported dissatisfaction. The higher figure for Scotland may again be due to the number of drug users from that locality. A total of 53 per cent of drug users (29 per cent of all those expressing dissatisfaction) had complaints to make about services from the voluntary sector.

The aspect of voluntary services which prompted the most comments (40) referred to the structure of the organisation and included concerns about the adequacy of funding, the expertise of volunteers, and the poor management of groups. The second area of dissatisfaction (20 respondents) concerned the overall atmosphere or ethics of the group and the extent to which people felt welcomed. A third concern was with the quality or structure of personal support (14 respondents). This category included poor experiences with 'buddies' and difficulties with relationships within a counselling setting. The fourth category of complaints included various 'gaps' perceived by respondents including insufficient services for families and young people, lack of venues or inadequate opening hours, and the need for people to help with practical skills.

A small number of respondents (15 per cent, 27 respondents) had approached a voluntary organisation and found help unavailable or unforthcoming. The most frequent assistance refused was financial. More often respondents reported instances of 'buck passing', groups proving difficult to contact or being unable to answer their specific queries.

Despite these complaints, the majority of voluntary service users felt the nature and quality of services provided was good and this was reflected in the importance placed on the role of peer group support and the number of people who preferred to use the voluntary sector. A total of 63 respondents (46 per cent) stated that there were services which they would prefer to obtain from the voluntary sector than from elsewhere. Their reasons referred to the better quality of counselling and personal support available from voluntary groups, a preference for peer group support and 'unbiased' information and advice. Respondents were also asked whether they had used a voluntary group because they believed that the help or service was unavailable from other sources. A high percentage (54 per cent) reported this to be the case, particularly in Scotland where the proportion was 83 per cent (Table 3.9).

The higher percentage shown for Scotland may be accounted for by the experiences of drug users. It was found that 58 per cent of drug users (23

Table 3.9 **Use of Voluntary Services Unavailable Elsewhere**

Area	No	%
London	34	57
Manchester	12	35
Scotland	25	83
Birmingham	2	18
National	74	54

respondents) had chosen to use a voluntary group because of the unavailability of services. The other services seen to be unavailable elsewhere were varied and included:

- welfare benefits advice and financial assistance (10 respondents)
- social and leisure activities (8 respondents)
- drug related advice and needle exchanges (7 respondents)
- 'buddies' and overnight carers (3 respondents)
- help with housing, transport (2 respondents)
- health maintenance (2 respondents)

Other Voluntary Sector Services

Over a third of the respondents (34 per cent) had made use of a telephone Helpline for information or advice concerning HIV/AIDS. The majority of Helpline users (60 per cent) had called once or twice, but a quarter of the users had rung several times and 10 per cent said that they rang Helplines regularly. The respondents had sought advice on a variety of matters including: how to contact local support groups, 'practical' advice, housing, legal issues, health problems, medication advice, safer sex, diet, welfare benefits and overseas travel. However, the most common reason for ringing a Helpline (31) was to receive emotional support and 'telephone counselling'. The respondents reported that in two-thirds of the calls they made (67 per cent) they had been happy with the advice received and considered the service to be satisfactory.

The respondents in this sample were asked additionally if they had participated in any conference or educational/training programmes organised via voluntary organisations and 64 respondents (35 per cent of the sample) had done so. The respondents from London had participated more in this type of activity (49 per cent) compared with Scotland (35 per cent), Manchester (23 per cent) and Birmingham (5 per cent) and the London respondents had made use of a wider variety of courses and conferences. The 64 respondents had attended a total of 71 such events between them which had been organised mainly via self-help or HIV specific voluntary groups.

3.4 Use of Social Services

This section examines the use of social services by people who are HIV positive and assesses the quality of service received.

Level of Contact with Social Services

Nearly half of the research sample (46 per cent, n=83) had seen a social worker since they were diagnosed antibody positive (Table 3.10).

Table 3.10 **Contact with Social Worker by Diagnosis**

Diagnosis	No.	% of Total Sample
HIV	34	32.1
ARC	23	65.7
AIDS	26	65.0
Total	**83**	**45.9**

Interestingly, fewer respondents from Manchester and Birmingham had seen a social worker (27 per cent and 5 per cent respectively), compared with respondents from London (56 per cent of the sample) and Scotland (74 per cent). This may in part be explained by the fact that a smaller percentage of respondents in the former two study areas had ARC and AIDS. Moreover, use of social services may not always be a consequence of HIV status. For example, in Scotland, social workers perform the role of probation officers, thus a proportion of Scottish drug users (n=15) will have had to use social services for this reason. Supply side factors such as ease of access to social services, and the existence of specialist services, for example, in some London boroughs, could also be relevant. It should be noted at this point that only 28 respondents (15 per cent of the sample) stated that they saw a social worker on a regular basis. The majority of respondents reporting to have had contact, had only seen a social worker on one or a few occasions, (n=55). Contact tended to be more regular for those respondents with ARC and AIDS.

Ninety eight respondents (54 per cent of the sample) had had no contact with social services at all since their diagnoses. The majority of these, 86 per cent (n=84) stated that they had no need for services available via social workers. A greater proportion of respondents with HIV stated that they did not need social work services—61 per cent of the sample. This compares with 29 per cent of respondents with ARC and 23 per cent of respondents with AIDS. Of the remaining respondents who had not seen a social worker, five stated that they had no information about services available or who to contact to access them; three stated that they felt threatened by social services/social work departments; and three felt that these services had not been made available to them.

When asked what type of social worker they had seen, 35 respondents stated that they had seen a general or area social worker (54 per cent of those in contact with social services). Thirty two respondents had seen a hospital social worker (38 per cent), and a further five (6 per cent) had seen a probation social worker. A greater percentage of respondents with AIDS (n=15, 38 per cent of those with AIDS) had had contact with hospital social services than respondents with HIV (n=10, 9 per cent of the sample).

As demonstrated in table 3.11 the major source of referral was via hospitals (56 per cent of referrals). Other medical routes, for example, via GPs were less well used (in six cases). In thirteen cases respondents self-referred. Self-referral was more common amongst respondents with HIV and ARC (n=6 respectively) compared with respondents with AIDS (n=1).

Table 3.11   **Routes of Referral to Social Services**

Referral Agency/Person	No.	Percent of Referrals
Hospital	48	55.8
Self	13	15.1
Voluntary Organisation/informal carers	10	11.6
Other medical	6	7.0
Housing	3	3.5
Other	6	7.0
Total	**86**	**100**

(Total number of respondents=83)

Reasons for Contact with Social Services

People approached social services for a number of reasons (see Table 3.12), the main one being for information and advice relating to benefits, housing and employment (35 per cent of reasons given by respondents to the survey). This reason was given by a greater proportion of respondents with AIDS than with ARC and HIV. In only 17 per cent of instances (n=16), did respondents want access to other social services and practical assistance. There was some variation by diagnosis, with respondents with ARC requiring this assistance in 25 per cent of instances (n=7) compared with respondents with AIDS (16 per cent of instances) and HIV (11 per cent). In 20 cases, respondents were referred to a social worker as a matter of routine. Other reasons for contact with social work services include respondents requiring financial help, needing support, rehabilitation and post-prison release.

Table 3.12   **Reasons for Seeking Social Services Assistance**

Reason	HIV (n=34)	ARC (n=23)	AIDS (n=26)	TOTAL (n=83)
Advice and Information	10	9	15	34
	(27.8)	(32.1)	(46.9)	(35.4)
Financial Help	3	3	3	9
	(8.3)	(10.7)	(9.4)	(9.4)
Access to Social Services/	4	7	5	16
Practical Help	(11.1)	(25.0)	(15.6)	(16.7)
Routine Referral	9	5	6	20
	(25.0)	(17.9)	(18.8)	(20.8)
Support	3	1	2	6
	(8.5)	(3.6)	(6.2)	(6.3)
Other[1]	7	3	1	11
	(19.5)	(10.7)	(3.1)	(11.4)

( ) figures in parenthesis=percentage of reasons expressed for contact(s) with social workers.

[1] Includes: after prison release, child in care, neighbours reported to SS, probation, rehabilitation, works at local drug group.

In 70 per cent of cases (n=58), the time which respondents had to wait before seeing a social worker was negligible. Eleven respondents reported that they had to wait up to a week, (14 per cent of those in contact), and only seven persons had to wait for two weeks or more. Seven respondents stated that delays in seeing a social worker caused them problems. These, however, were not specified.

Of the 83 people who had contact with a social worker, 69 (83 per cent) reported that a social worker had arranged particular services for them or had acted as an intermediary in gaining access to services. There was considerable variation by study locality with 90 per cent of respondents in Scotland having had services arranged for them, compared with 58 per cent of those in London, 25 per cent of those in Manchester and 5 per cent in Birmingham. Table 3.13 summarises assistance arranged or facilitated by social workers according to diagnosis.

Table 3.13 **Services Arranged by Social Workers, by Diagnosis**

Service	HIV (n=26)	ARC (n=22)	AIDS (n=21)	TOTAL (n=69)
Practical Assistance	10 (33.3)	16 (50.0)	16 (54.3)	42 (47.2)
Financial/Benefits Advice and Help	11 (36.7)	9 (28.1)	8 (29.6)	28 (31.5)
General Advice and Support	8 (26.7)	6 (18.8)	1 (3.7)	15 (16.8)
Health/Information/ Advice/Referral	1 (3.3)	1 (3.1)	2 (7.4)	4 (4.5)

Respondents with ARC and AIDS were more likely to have received practical help, which took the form of help with rehousing, receiving bus or travel passes and home help services.

In addition to these services, 34 respondents (41 per cent of those in contact with a social worker) had services arranged which they had not specifically requested. There was a greater proportion of people with AIDS receiving these additional services. The majority of those who expressed an opinion on these unrequested services (54 per cent) said they were happy with the arrangements or felt they had received positive support. However, 46 per cent said they were either displeased, or had mixed feelings because they felt that they did not require the service provided.

As well as providing services, social workers were also able to refer people to other service providers as appropriate; 22 respondents reported that they had been referred in this way. There were 11 referrals to health services, nine to other social service departments, three to housing advice organisations and four to voluntary organisations (and two to unspecified agencies).

Respondents were referred on for practical help (n=8), advice (n=8), health related services (n=7) and financial help (n=4).

The Question of Disclosure

In 79 cases (95 per cent of those in contact with a social worker), social workers were aware of the respondent's antibody status. Only 22 respondents (28 per cent) had informed their social worker of their status themselves. In the remaining cases social workers had been informed by social services staff or health personnel or by other persons. It is not known whether this was done with the respondents consent. As many as 16 respondents did not know how their social worker had been informed which implies a lack of consent and, possibly, breach of confidentiality.

Quality of Service

In general the services provided by social workers were considered to be helpful, particularly financial assistance and advice, general advice and counselling and practical assistance. At least one social work service was found helpful by 53 respondents (64 per cent). However 30 respondents (36 per cent) had one or more complaints about their contact with social work staff, including general dissatisfaction with social work services, problems associated with breach of confidentiality and delays in receiving assistance.

Respondents were asked to give their opinions, based on their personal experience or on their knowledge of others' experiences, on a number of statements regarding social services. Statements and a summary of respondents' views are shown in Table 3.14.

These responses include people who have had personal contact with social workers and those who have not. Significantly users of the service were more likely to express positive opinions than those without. Table 3.15 gives a breakdown of those agreeing with each statement according to whether they had the personal experience of social work services.

People with a personal experience of social services had a more favourable opinion of the quality of service than had non-users, showing a relatively high expectation among non-users that the service would be unsatisfactory.

Table 3.14 **Respondents' Views on Social Services**

Statement	Strongly Agree	Agree	No Opinion	Disagree	Strongly Disagree	Other	No. of responses
Social workers are good at providing practical help	10 (7)	82 (59)	9 (7)	26 (19)	8 (6)	3 (2)	138
Social workers are good at providing emotional support	7 (5)	47 (34)	19 (14)	49 (36)	13 (10)	1 (1)	136
Social workers take your own wishes into account	7 (5)	81 (59)	11 (8)	30 (22)	7 (5)	1 (1)	137
Social workers consult you before changing plans or arrangements	7 (5)	54 (40)	32 (24)	32 (24)	10 (7)	— (—)	135
Social workers are good at keeping things in confidence	15 (12)	51 (39)	34 (26)	20 (15)	9 (7)	1 (1)	130

(1) percentage of those expressing an opinion

Table 3.15 **Respondents' Views on Social Work Services According to Personal Experience**

	Percentage of users agreeing or strongly agreeing	Percentage of non-users agreeing or strongly agreeing	Average Percentage
Social workers are good at providing practical help	75	55	66
Social workers are good at providing emotional support	48	29	39
Social workers take your own needs and wishes into account	71	53	64
Social workers are good at keeping things in confidence	57	35	51

3.5 Use of Health Services

The focus of this book is the demand for and supply of social care for people with HIV, ARC or AIDS with an emphasis on how to enable people to remain in the community, but there is a considerable overlap between social care and health care in respect of HIV infection. For this reason the respondents in this sample were asked a series of questions concerning their use of health services: primary care, out-patient services, in-patient services, health services in the home and dentistry to determine the extent and nature of use, the level of satisfaction with the services received or on offer, and whether use of these services imposed any financial cost on the individual.

Outpatient Services

Only six of the 181 respondents in this sample (3 per cent) stated that they were not in contact with an out-patient department and five of these six respondents (none of whom had ARC or AIDS) had been originally tested at a hospital clinic—the sixth person having been tested via his/her GP. The remaining 175 respondents reported a wide use of hospital out-patient departments which include one-off visits to an HIV-related clinic, regular check-ups at clinics, and occasional visits to specialist departments in respect of particular health disorders.

A total of 65 respondents (37 per cent of out-patient users) reported experiencing one or more problems with their use of out-patient services. The most common problem faced by these respondents (46 comments) concerned the physical or emotional difficulties encountered in visiting hospital departments. Where the respondents were experiencing illness, mobility problems or fatigue (18) the journey to out-patient departments, the length of the visit, or the examinations required entailed physical discomfort. A further 28 respondents described the emotional difficulties that they faced during out-patient visits with tension, embarrassment and feelings of vulnerability being mentioned. Meeting other people with the virus, perhaps on a regular basis was often described as 'depressing' particularly where one witnessed, over time, a worsening of their condition. Where the out-patient visit entailed a regular blood test, for example, a cell count, the respondents often experienced feelings of anxiety and apprehension at the potential prospect of 'bad news'. A typical comment which illustrates this experience was that the respondent felt acutely depressed for a number of days prior to his appointment, having to combat his fears concerning a possible rediagnosis of his condition. This stress then resulted in a further period of fatigue following the appointment.

A further 28 comments referred to problems concerning inconvenience and confidentiality. The difficulties posed by inconvenient appointment times and the unavailability of consultations outside of working hours (evenings and weekends) were mentioned by 11 respondents. Long waiting times at the clinics were mentioned by six people and the difficulties imposed by a lack of transport or the distance between home and hospital were reported by five respondents. A further six respondents described experiencing problems with confidentiality where, for example, they sat in waiting rooms of clinics known to be used for people with HIV-AIDS, meeting other people with the virus, or having to conceal their HIV status from members of hospital staff. Other comments (11) were in the nature of complaints concerning the clinics or the staff; receiving differing opinions from different clinics or consultants (5); a lack of information from doctors (3); having to mix with drug users (1); a 'conveyor belt' attitude (1) and 'inefficiency' (1 respondent). Problems with or complaints about out-patient services were more frequently expressed by Scottish respondents (55 per cent of users) compared with London (43 per cent), Manchester (29 per cent) and Birmingham (5 per cent).

A small majority of the respondents (54 per cent) usually visited the out-patient clinic on their own. A total of 22 respondents (13 per cent) said that they were always accompanied by someone else, and 56 respondents (32 per cent) said that they sometimes took someone with them. Therefore the costs of out-patient visits in terms of time and travel fall not only upon the 78 respondents. The respondents were asked who they chose to accompany them and ten out of the 78 respondents varied their companions according to circumstances. In only a few cases were respondents accompanied by members of the statutory or voluntary sector and friends and partners performed the role of companion most frequently.

The reason why respondents chose to be accompanied was not always known. However, the emotional stress experienced by a number of respondents attending out-patient clinics is underlined by the fact that in 47 per cent of cases the respondent chose to be accompanied for 'moral support' or 'reassurance' rather than for practical assistance. In 10 per cent of cases the respondent chose to go with either a partner or an HIV positive friend because it was 'convenient' to arrange appointment times which coincided. In 16 per cent of cases the respondent required assistance either with walking, transport, a wheelchair, or in case of illness.

A total of 74 respondents (42 per cent of those using out-patient departments) stated that they had been referred by the department for help or treatment elsewhere; 48 respondents cited one referral, 14 respondents cited two referrals and 12 respondents gave details of three referrals totalling 112 referrals for the total sample. Those people with ARC or AIDS were more likey to have been directed towards other services (67 per cent and 53 per cent respectively) compared with 30 per cent of people who were HIV positive. The respondents from London had been referred elsewhere more frequently (61 per cent) compared with Scotland (45 per cent) and Manchester (24 per cent). None of the Birmingham respondents reported a referral. In 79 per cent of cases the referral was for other medical or specialist treatment from, for example, a dermatologist, a neurologist or surgeon. Respondents in London were more frequently referred for medical or specialist treatment. In 11 per cent of cases the referral was for psychiatric support or treatment. London respondents were least likely to receive such referrals. Two respondents were referred to a social worker; two to a voluntary organisation, and one to a general practitioner.

Table 3.16 **Respondents' Views on Outpatient Services**

	Strongly agree	Agree	Disagree	Strongly Disagree	No/or Varied Opinion
	%	%	%	%	%
O/P depts are good at providing practical help	8	62	24	1	5
O/P depts are good at providing emotional support	7	39	40	5	9
The staff take your own needs and wishes into account	9	65	19	2	5
The staff consult you before changing plans/arrangements	8	63	17	3	9
The staff are good at keeping things in confidence	10	69	5	1	15

All the respondents were asked about their pattern of out-patient treatment since having the virus. As might be anticipated, 93 per cent of the sample said that they had visited out-patient departments more since knowing they were antibody positive.

The respondents were asked to comment on a series of statements regarding certain aspects of out-patient services and 172 respondents gave their views (Table 3.16).

The quality of 'emotional support' provided by out-patient departments and their staff was therefore questioned by a substantial number of the respondents. However, out-patient departments appeared, from these opinions, to be taking regard of confidentiality issues. The respondents in Manchester expressed disagreement with the above statements most often. With the lowest 'positive' scores in all but the fourth statement, where Scottish respondents expressed most disagreement.

Inpatient Care

A total of 83 respondents (46 per cent of the sample) had been admitted to a hospital ward 'because of the virus'. Scottish respondents had experienced inpatient stays more frequently (65 per cent) compared with respondents from London (47 per cent), Manchester (40 per cent) and Birmingham (26 per cent). The drug users in this survey were more likely to have been in-patients: 55 per cent of drug users compared with 43 per cent of non-drug users. As might be anticipated, a higher percentage of people with ARC or AIDS had been inpatients (66 per cent and 95 per cent respectively) but it was found also that 21 per cent of people who were HIV positive had also been in hospital. The respondents were invited to describe up to three inpatient stays and from these data it was found that 34 respondents had one hospital stay; 23 respondents had two stays, 26 respondents had three stays, totalling 158 reported stays, the majority of these stays (84 per cent) had taken place during the period of this study, that is between 1988 and 1990.

Respondents provided details of the reasons for their admittance to hospital and the duration of each stay. The most frequent reason for being admitted (41 per cent) was a respiratory disorder, for example, PCP, pneumonia, tuberculosis and 'chest infections' of which PCP was the most common illness reported.

When asked whether, apart from the obvious distress caused through illness, their stay in hospital had caused them any particular personal problems, 37 respondents (45 per cent of inpatients) cited specific emotional distress that they experienced whilst in hospital and especially feelings of 'isolation'. Worries concerning their home and housing were mentioned by nine per cent of the respondents, one of whom had been evicted whilst in hospital. A further nine per cent of problems related to practical aspects of being a patient in hospital, including transport to hospital, bureaucracy and 'paperwork', inconvenient visiting hours or a preference for a private ward. A total of eight per cent of respondents mentioned the distressing aspects of particular treatments and a further eight per cent described financial worries, for example, having benefits stopped whilst in hospital and having no money to buy soap or other items for their hospital stay. Problems and worries concerning employment were reported by six per cent of the respondents, including the problem of being on an AIDS ward whilst concealing one's HIV status from employers and colleagues. Confidentiality problems and staff attitudes were mentioned by three per cent of the respondents and included, for example, one respondent who had been 'rejected' by hospital staff.

Some of the above concerns overlapped the responses given by the respondents when asked whether they had considered any of the inpatient services to be unsatisfactory. A total of 38 respondents (46 per cent of inpatients) had one or more complaints to make about their stay in hospital:

- ward/hospital regime (29 per cent) for example, lack of communication between staff and patient; delays; 'authoritarian' regimes; 'conveyor-belt' attitudes.

- conditions (27 per cent) for example, 'inedible' food, noisy wards;

- segregation (23 per cent) for example, hostile staff attitudes; segregated facilities; over-cautious or inappropriate infection control (staff in protective clothing); staff 'insensitivity';

- treatment (16 per cent) for example, 'poor' or 'inadequate' medical care; 'inexperienced' doctors; poor knowledge of HIV-AIDS;

- other (5 per cent) for example, lack of stimulation for patients, particularly for longer-term patients.

Respondents who had been inpatients were also invited to describe those aspects of inpatient care which had been particularly pleasing and 78 per cent of the people who had been patients (65 respondents) gave one or more examples. The 'caring' qualities of hospital staff were referred to by the majority of these respondents (51 comments) who felt that either all staff or particular staff had been especially supportive, helpful or understanding. Nurses were singled out most frequently for their caring attitudes but other staff were mentioned also, particularly consultants, hospital chaplains and dieticians. The provision of 'counselling' support by hospital staff was welcomed by ten respondents and a further 14 respondents felt that conditions and facilities on the ward had been especially satisfactory, for example, having televisions, a home support team to discuss future care, and the privacy of a separate room.

On this latter point, the decision whether or not to provide separate facilities for inpatients with the virus is complex. These interviews suggest that where some people had been given a private room they had felt themselves to be receiving discriminatory treatment and spoke of 'segregation', whilst others welcomed the fact that they had additional privacy. Clearly where patients are segregated against their wishes or because of unfounded concern over infection control, there is a cause for concern. In the majority of hospitals around the country there will be no separate AIDS ward and inpatients are most likely to be admitted to an Infectious Diseases or similar ward. Depending on the design of the local facilities, such wards may be multi-bedded or contain a mix of, for example, 4–6 bed and 1-bed units. In such circumstances it is not unusual for more seriously ill patients to be accommodated separately. Problems may arise, however, where accommodation in a separate ward is, in itself, interpreted by other patients or hospital staff as an indication that the patient 'had AIDS' with the resulting implications for confidentiality. Whilst hospital staff should be receiving training concerning the possibility of working with HIV-AIDS patients, it is not known whether private contractors working within the NHS are training staff adequately and such potential loopholes in systems of confidentiality need to be considered.

In addition to the above questions relating to people's direct experiences on the wards, the respondents were questioned regarding some of the more practical aspects of inpatient services. Firstly, they were asked whether, in their opinion, they thought that any of the services could have been provided in the home. Only 11 of the respondents felt this to be the case and gave examples of particular treatments or advice, for example, the services of nutritionists, physiotherapists and occupational therapists, check-ups and 'monitoring'.

Respondents were asked whether they felt that their stays in hospital had ever been prolonged because of home circumstances. A total of 14 respondents believed that they could have been discharged earlier or could have prevented hospital admission had it not been for their home or housing circumstances. The most common problem reported (nine respondents) was having no-one at home to look after them and the other five respondents reported being homeless or having unsuitable accommodation (for example, Bed and Breakfast accommodation).

A total of 22 respondents (27 per cent of inpatients) described facing problems following their discharge from hospital). The most common problem (12 respondents) referred to the individual's health state or mobility. In none of the cases where respondents faced pain or immobility did they receive assistance from formal sources of support but rather they 'coped' alone or with the help of friends, for example:

- respondents could not manage the stairs so slept on the floor downstairs;

- respondent needed crutches when leaving hospital but was told none were available;

- a single parent had difficulty coping with the needs of a young child whilst still unwell;

- friends helped with decorating and furnishing new home.

A further seven respondents spoke of problems with housing or housing costs following hospital discharge, for example, returning home to find the house had been neglected; needing to be rehoused; or facing accumulated bills. Another three respondents mentioned the emotional impact of illness following their in-patient stay, for example, having to face a new diagnosis. Whilst the number of respondents facing problems was small they represent over a quarter of all those with experience of inpatient services.

It was found that only a minority of people having treatment on a hospital ward (37 per cent, 31 respondents) had had any discussion concerning their home circumstances prior to their discharge. Where staff had enquired as to the patient's circumstances, this was either medical staff (eight respondents), social workers and members of a Home Support Team (eight respondents), hospital 'counsellors' (four respondents) or other staff. In 23 of the 31 cases, advice or practical assistance was provided as a result of

these pre-discharge discussions such as help with re-housing, the organisation of informal support, discussions with family/partners, ensuring that
accommodation was suitable for mobility needs, and so forth. It is possible,
depending on the nature of illness and the impact upon mobility, that medical staff or hospital based social workers may not anticipate problems for
some patients. However, throughout this survey there have been a proportion of respondents who face housing difficulties or problems with coping
emotionally irrespective of the degree of illness they have experienced. This
survey has also shown that not all people with the virus may have well-
developed networks of informal support on which to rely and therefore
hospital and social services staff cannot assume that such care will always
be available.

The respondents were asked to comment on five statements to ascertain
their opinion of inpatient services and 168 respondents replied. Table 3.17
shows, therefore, the total responses of this sample and includes the opinions of people who had not been inpatients. When these data were analysed
for 'users' and 'non-users' of inpatient services (Table 3.17), there was a

Table 3.17   **Respondents' Views on Inpatient Care**

	Strongly Agree	Agree	Disagree	Strongly Disagree	No/or Varied Opinion
	%	%	%	%	%
Hospital wards are good at providing practical help	5	62	10	2	21
Hospital wards are good at providing emotional support	7	43	22	5	23
The staff take your own needs and wishes into account	5	53	14	3	25
The staff consult you before changing plans/ arrangements	5	44	21	4	26
The staff are good at keeping things in confidence	7	60	8	1	24

Table 3.18   **Users' and Non Users' Views on Inpatient Care**

	% of Users who Agreed/ Strongly Agreed	% of Non-Users who Agreed/Strongly Agreed
Hospital wards are good at providing practical help	86	57
Hospital wards are good at providing emotional support	65	36
The staff take your own needs and wishes into account	76	43
The staff consult you before changing plans/ arrangements	66	34
The staff are good at keeping things in confidence	80	55

marked difference of opinion with users showing consistently higher levels of agreement with the statements. These findings reveal a low expectation of satisfaction with inpatient services amongst those who have not been admitted to hospital. The highest levels of agreement with these statements were from Scottish respondents who included a higher proportion of 'users' of inpatient care. The highest level of disagreement came from Birmingham respondents who included a higher proportion of 'non-users'. Discounting these Birmingham results, London respondents scored the highest levels of disagreement/dissatisfaction.

The number of people who had no opinion reflects the higher number of non-users of inpatient, compared with out-patient services.

Health Services in the Home

Only 18 respondents (10 per cent of the sample) had received medical or health-related care in their home (other than primary care) and this was most likely to have been the case for people with ARC or AIDS (17 per cent and 20 per cent respectively) compared with people who are HIV positive (4 per cent). Table 3.19 shows the health services received by these respondents.

Table 3.19   **Health Services in the Home**

	No. of Respondents[1]
Home support team	7
District nurse/nurse/health visitor	7
Consultant/hospital doctor	2
Occupational therapist	2
Specialist nurse eg, drugs team, haemophilia	2
Community psychiatric nurse	1
'Counsellor'	1

[1] three respondents received visits from more than one person.

In only a minority of instances was the visit reported as being associated with direct medical 'treatment' with the majority of visits being to provide 'support' or to monitor how the individual was coping at home (13). Other visits were to provide medications/injections (4), medical examinations/checkups (4), dressings (1) and help with bathing (1). Only three people reported experiencing a problem with health care in the home: a district nurse refused to touch the respondent; post-operative support was insufficient; and promised assistance was not forthcoming.

The respondents were asked whether there were any health services they would like to see provided in the home, but which are not at present available to them and 28 respondents (15 per cent of the sample) gave one or more examples. A total of 12 respondents did not specify the type of help they required, but felt generally that more treatment should be available in the community to prevent hospitalisation. Other respondents were more specific regarding treatments, for example, blood transfusions, nebulisers, pentamidine (5) whilst others referred to health-related services such as physiotherapy, chiropody, massage and occupational therapy (6). A further five respondents wished to have their health monitored at home rather than having to visit outpatient departments and one respondent mentioned the need for day and night carers.

The respondents were asked to give their opinion on five statements concerning these services. However because of the small number of 'users' it is more appropriate to consider the differences of opinion between 'users' and 'non-users' rather than the overall sample responses (Table 3.20). There was a greater consensus of opinion on these services compared with out and

Table 3.20   **Respondents' Views on Health Services Provided at Home**

Medical staff who visit the home:	% of Users Who Agreed/ Strongly Agreed	% of non-users Who Agreed/Strongly Agreed
are good at providing practical help	56	69
are good at providing emotional support	56	42
take your own needs and wishes into account	61	68
consult you before changing plans/arrangements	56	53
are good at keeping things in confidence	56	58

inpatient services but interestingly, on the question of practical help, individual needs and confidentiality, the non-users had a higher expectation of satisfaction.

Quality of Hospital Services

The respondents were given the opportunity to discuss any problems that they had experienced with hospital services overall (that is, in the home, in-patient care and out-patient services) which they had not previously mentioned. A total of 60 respondents had one or more specific concerns or complaints which they wished to raise. The largest category of complaints (20 respondents) referred to the overall standard or organisation of hospital services and included complaints concerning overcrowded or 'over-worked' departments (12); underfunding (4); negative attitudes towards people with HIV-AIDS (3); and the varying quality of care between hospitals (one respondent). The second largest category of complaints (15 respondents) centred on the respondents' opinions of medical staff and included complaints that staff were inadequately trained to provide emotional support (6); that there was a lack of communication between doctor/hospital and patient (6); staff inexperience with HIV-AIDS (2); and one respondent felt that services were motivated by research, rather than patient needs. The availability of services was mentioned by seven respondents who commented on: the frequency of staff changes making relationships difficult (3); the unavailability of doctors at weekends (2); the need for emergency access or an on-call system (1) and a general difficulty in gaining access to medical care (1). A number of respondents (10) also wished to describe personal difficulties they had experienced which included breaches of confidentiality, a lack of respite care (especially for people with children), the problem of moving clinics and being re-examined, poor treatment, and the intolerance of medical staff towards unorthodox medicine. The overall level of satisfaction with hospital services as illustrated by the reaction of respondents to the five statements shown previously appears to be high with an average of 20 per cent of respondents expressing dissatisfaction. However, there is some consensus that emotional support is less satisfactory.

Medical care for people with HIV-AIDS is most often organised via specialist hospital services, consultants or clinics and specialised HIV-AIDS units. Similar facilities based in hospitals may be used as the focus of medical support for patients from a wide area. The role of general practitioners in respect of medical care for people with HIV-AIDS is, to date, far more limited with the possible exception of those GPs involved in the direct care of drug users.

Primary Care

Respondents were asked whether they were registered with a local doctor and 156 of the 181 respondents had a general practitioner (86 per cent of the sample). It was found that 17 per cent of London respondents, 16 per cent of Brirmingham, 12 per cent of Manchester, and three per cent of Scottish respondents were not registered with a GP. The respondents were further asked whether their local doctor was aware that they had the virus. One-third of the sample (60 respondents) said that their doctor did not know of their HIV status. The Birmingham respondents were least likely to have informed a GP (58 per cent) compared with 40 per cent in Manchester, 33 per cent in London and three per cent in Scotland. These figures are higher than anticipated, and they should also be seen in the context that 31 per cent of people with ARC and 30 percent of people with AIDS did not have a GP who was aware of their HIV status. From the findings of this survey it is clear that there may be many general practitioners who believe that they do not have HIV-AIDS patients when, in fact, they do.

When the respondents were asked about their use of primary care, 130 people (72 per cent) stated that they had seen a GP since knowing that they had the virus. Despite the fact that a high proportion of doctors did not know their patient's status, in only a very few cases did the respondent state that he/she had presented with health problems unrelated to HIV infection, for example, hay fever and injuries. It was found that 78 per cent of drug users, compared with 67 per cent of non-drug users had seen a local doctor.

Those people who had not seen a local doctor were asked why and 14 of the 51 respondents stated that they had 'no need'. A further 27 respondents said that all of their requirements for health care were catered for by an 'HIV clinic', negating their need to either register with or use a general practitioner. Another nine respondents stated that they were deterred from using a GP because they felt the doctor was insufficiently informed about HIV-AIDS.

Over a quarter of the sample (28 per cent) had changed their general practitioner since knowing that they had the virus and this had most frequently occurred in Scotland (45 per cent) compared with London (35 per cent) and Manchester (15 per cent). Just one person from Birmingham had changed their doctor. These 50 respondents had changed their GP for various reasons, not all of which were related to their HIV status. For example, people had moved to other areas, or doctors had moved or retired and this left 18 people who had changed their doctor for reasons concerning their HIV status.

- eight respondents felt that their original GP knew little about HIV-AIDS or was unsympathetic to their status;

- five people had been refused treatment by their original GP, because of either their HIV status or their drug use;

- three respondents who were drug-users felt that the treatment they received was inappropriate for their withdrawal symptoms;

- two respondents had changed doctors for confidentiality reasons: one to seek a doctor outside of his/her locality and one because of the lack of confidentiality within the practice.

All the respondents were asked whether they had experienced any difficulty in finding or using a general practitioner and 50 people (28 per cent of the sample) said that they had. It was found that 41 of these respondents had informed their doctor of their HIV status. The 50 respondents gave one or more examples of problems that they had encountered. The most common problem concerned the 'attitude' of the doctor towards a patient who was HIV positive or a drug-user (23 respondents) and included comments such as, 'the doctor was panic stricken'. 'the doctor said he/she needed Health Service clearance to treat me'. Other respondents felt that they had been neglected, with doctors unwilling to make home visits or to physically examine the patient. Two respondents had been informed that because of the changes in GP budgeting they were now considered 'expensive' patients.

A total of 16 respondents complained of receiving unsatisfactory medical care because the doctor was inexperienced in HIV-AIDS, and 11 respondents had met difficulty in finding a GP who was willing to treat them. Two respondents needed the assistance of a hospital and a social worker to find a 'sympathetic' doctor. A further six respondents had been refused acceptance onto a doctor's list because of their HIV status. In nine cases the respondents complained about the lack of continuity of doctors (for example, where locums were employed), surgery waiting times, the problems caused by having to pay for 'sick notes' and the embarrassment of facing a doctor they had known for many years.

When asked whether their use of general practitioners had changed since knowing that they had the virus, the respondents replied as shown in Table 3.21.

Table 3.21 **Changes in Use of General Practitioner**

Changes in Use	Number	Per Cent
Much more	24	13
A bit more	26	14
No change	70	39
A bit less	16	9
Much less	38	21
Not known	7	4
Total	**181**	**100**

A total of 153 respondents gave their responses to the five statements in respect of general practitioner services and only in the case of 'confidentiality' did a majority of the respondents agree with the statements (Table 3.22). The highest level of dissatisfaction (two-thirds of the respondents) was with the level of emotional support.

It was found that people who had used a GP since knowing that they had the virus were more likely to agree with the above statements revealing a high expectation amongst non-users that GP services would be unsatisfactory (Table 3.23).

104

Table 3.22   **Respondents' Views on General Practitioner Services**

	Strongly Agree	Agree	Disagree	Strongly Disagree	No/or Varied Opinion
	%	%	%	%	%
Local Drs are good at providing practical help	3	41	41	10	5
Local Drs are good at providing emotional support	3	23	46	20	8
Local Drs take your own needs and wishes into account	4	40	35	8	13
Local Drs consult you before changing plans/ arrangements	3	42	23	5	27
Local Drs are good at keeping things in confidence	5	57	11	3	24

Table 3.23   **Respondents' Views on GP Services, by Use**

	% of Users who Agreed/ Strongly Agreed	% of Non-Users who Agreed/Strongly Agreed
Local Drs are good at providing practical help	52	22
Local Drs are good at providing emotional support	30	15
Local Drs take your own needs and wishes into account	50	29
Local Drs consult you before changing plans/ arrangements	47	39
Local Drs are good at keeping things in confidence	70	36

Dental Services

Respondents were asked whether they had visited a dentist since knowing that they had the virus. It was found that 71 per cent of the sample (128 respondents) had seen a dentist of which 81 respondents (45 per cent of the sample) had visited a local dentist and 47 respondents (26 per cent of the sample) had received dental treatment from 'private' sources, hospital clinics or dental hospitals. The reasons why people had not visited a dentist were unknown in seven cases but the remaining 46 respondents replied as follows:

- no need for dental treatment (35 respondents)
- 'putting it off' (4 respondents)
- would be/have been refused treatment (3 respondents)
- 'no point' given current poor state of health (2 respondents)
- cannot afford treatment (2 respondents).

It was found that 24 respondents (13 per cent of the sample) had been refused dental treatment because of their HIV status, including one respondent who had been refused treatment whilst in prison and another who was told he would only be given treatment if he paid. A further eight respondents described receiving treatment under distressing circumstances, for example, being seen only in a hut away from the dental surgery, having bleach sprayed throughout the surgery, having all equipment covered in cling-film, and being made to collect and clear up his/her sputum. Another two respondents said that they had only been treated because they agreed to an appointment 'at the end of the day' which was inconvenient and made them feel stigmatised.

A total of 59 respondents had changed their dentist since knowing that they had the virus (33 per cent of the sample). In 41 of the 59 instances of change the reasons had been associated with the respondent's HIV status and included those who had been refused treatment or who had received unsatisfactory treatment. A further four respondents had changed their dentist because of problems concerning confidentiality and 16 of the 41 respondents had been recommended to other dentists or clinics which were willing to accept HIV-AIDS patients.

3.6 Use of private services

Respondents were asked if they had paid for any services since knowing they had the virus. This section looks at a variety of practical and medical private services used by respondents, and examines why respondents chose to pay for them.

Practical Services

It was found that only a small proportion of the sample, 14 respondents (eight per cent), had paid for practical services in the home. Eleven of these were London respondents, (14 per cent of the London sample). Table 3.24 shows the types of private services used.

Table 3.24   **Use of Private Services: Practical Help at Home**

Services[1]	No. of Respondents
Cleaning	6
Painting and decorating	3
Moving	2
Repairs	2
Window cleaning	2

[1] Other services used by only one person include steam cleaning of upholstery, moving furniture and gardening.

Few respondents used the services on a regular basis. In most cases, (63 per cent of instances) practical private services had only been used on one or two occasions.

In 12 of the 14 cases, respondents sought private services for reasons related to their antibody status, ie, fatigue and not being able to undertake tasks themselves because of the virus. One person had been refused cleaning services due to their antibody status.

Special Treatment and Therapies

A total of 28 respondents (15 per cent of the sample) reported that they had paid for special treatments and therapies to promote their physical and psychological well-being. It was found that while these respondents varied little in terms of diagnosis, there were considerable differences in terms of study locality. The vast majority of those paying for special treatments were

London respondents—25 persons (31 per cent of the London sample), compared with two Manchester respondents and nine in both Scotland and Birmingham. These figures may reflect the more widespread availability of less orthodox forms of treatments in London.

Sixteen different therapies and special treatments were reported to be used by respondents with 11 persons paying for two or more treatments. The most popular were massage (39 per cent of total), acupuncture (32 per cent), homeopathy (21 per cent) and aromatherapy (14 per cent).

In contrast with practical services in the home, respondents used private therapies and treatments on a regular basis in 43 per cent of cases.

In the vast majority of instances, private therapy/treatments were used because of the virus and HIV-related reasons (85 per cent of instances). Fifteen respondents identified reasons why services were helpful to them: in many cases simply because they 'worked' for the individuals concerned. Seven respondents found some treatments unsatisfactory, mainly because they were expensive.

When asked why they were willing to pay for special treatments and therapies, 18 respondents (64 per cent of those using such services) stated that they paid because the sorts of treatments were not available from statutory health services providers. A further two persons stated that they did not know where these services were available without charge. Some voluntary organisations provide or organise 'alternative' therapies for people with the virus, but these are not always free of charge.

Private Medical Schemes

Only 18 respondents belonged to private medical schemes (10 per cent of the sample). Of these, the majority were London respondents (78 per cent) and 16 of the 18 had joined schemes before they were known to be HIV positive.

Half of the respondents (n=9) stated that they had made the decision to join a scheme themselves, with the other half (n=9) joining as part of their conditions of employment.

Only seven respondents (five with AIDS and two with HIV), recorded having used private medical schemes since their diagnosis. A further person was apprehensive of using the scheme lest this should lead to work colleagues discovering his/her status.

Private Medical Treatment

Eleven respondents stated that they had paid for private medical treatment, four people on more than one occasion. In six instances, this occurred when the respondent was abroad. Only one respondent had been refused medical treatment.

Reasons for choosing to pay for treatment included needing a doctor immediately (in five cases), and dissatisfaction with the NHS (in four cases).

4 Organisation and Costs of Service Components:
Applying the Social Care Supply Framework (SCSF)

Overview

To examine the local authority organisational/policy response to HIV-AIDS, data were collected from the SSD/SWDs, housing, education and enviromental health departments of each of the five local authorities. These data were supplemented by information from 65 SSD/SWDs which participated in a national (ie, England, Scotland and Wales) survey of HIV-AIDS related social care supply patterns and plans, and by information derived from questionnaires completed by 102 voluntary agencies based in and around the study localities. Aggregate cost estimates were made for the five local authorities only.

This chapter outlines the use of the Social Care Supply Framework for the analysis of the service supply response of the five authorities in the study. This demonstrated that each was involved in a wide variety of HIV-AIDS related services initiatives, either through the use of special programmes and/or the use of existing services. Nonetheless, HIV-AIDS service planning had largely been undertaken without a clear and ordered framework within which to assess the organisational and cost consequences on an authority-wide basis. The SCSF provides an explicit and logical framework with which to attempt this.

4.1 Management and Coordination

HIV Coordinators in the Five Study authorities

All five study authorities have established specific lead, coordinating posts in respect of HIV-AIDS but there is considerable variation in the precise management arrangements. Nevertheless, job descriptions are similar and encompass coordination, liaison with other statutory and voluntary organisations and service development. An indication of the centrality of liaison work is provided by the fact that the officers refer to themselves as 'coordinators'—even though the word does not appear in their job titles.

Liaison and coordination work is given great emphasis both in job descriptions and HIV-AIDS Coordinators' accounts of their priorities and work.

Reticulist skills are required for the development of inter-organisational relationships and the need for such skills was certainly emphasised by HIV-AIDS Coordinators and others.

In their search for a rapid organisational response to the HIV-AIDS issue, three authorities, Hammersmith and Fulham, Kensington and Chelsea and Lothian, opted for the well-established Principal Officer model. The earliest appointment (October 1985) was in Hammersmith and Fulham. Lothian and Kensington and Chelsea did not appoint until January 1988 and February 1988 respectively. In each of these three authorities, the formal title of the HIV-AIDS Coordinator is Principal Officer HIV-AIDS. The appointee in Lothian SWD was originally described as an AIDS Advisor.

Not all the Principal Officers HIV-AIDS have a local authority background and there is evidence to suggest that the absence of such a background can create difficulties. In Lothian, the Principal Officer HIV-AIDS came from a voluntary drug/AIDS agency funded by the Health Board, and whilst his background is appropriate in many ways, the incumbent has had to adapt to a very different organisational culture. In contrast, the Principal Officer HIV-AIDS in Hammersmith and Fulham was a Community Social Worker and shop steward and became involved in the HIV-AIDS area because of discrimination against an employee who was HIV positive. This, together with two cases where home helps refused to provide care to people with AIDS, led to his present appointment. Thus, the Principal Officer HIV-AIDS in Hammersmith and Fulham not only came from a local authority back-ground but from the local authority in which he was appointed. Some of the rapid service development was clearly helped by this.

Manchester did not appoint a Principal Officer HIV-AIDS. In Manchester, an AIDS Unit was established in June 1987 at the suggestion of an AIDS Working Party. It was staffed by secondees from other local authority departments. From the beginning, Manchester's approach to the HIV-AIDS issue has been to emphasise the need for an authority-wide response. The creation of a central unit, staffed by secondees from a number of departments, reflects this perception. A conscious decision was taken not to base the unit in the Social Services Department in order to avoid the impression that HIV-AIDS had no implications for other local authority departments. The HIV-AIDS Coordinator in Manchester occupies a qualitatively different role from those performed by the Principal Officers in Hammersmith and Fulham, Kensington and Chelsea and Lothian. Organisationally, he occupies a much more strategic position and is responsible for corporate rather than departmental strategy.

Westminster fits neither the Principal Officer HIV-AIDS model nor the 'corporate coordinator' model found in Manchester. In Westminster, the most important central post is that of the Assistant Divisional Director (Disability and Health) in whom responsibility for HIV-AIDS is vested. Her job description notes that 25 per cent of her time is allocated to HIV-AIDS but the proportion of her time devoted to this area appears to be more in the order of 50 per cent. There is a large 'gap' between the Assistant Divisional Director (Disability and Health) and borough services consisting of specialist community/domiciliary care teams. The Community Care Team Leader has, however, an informal though recognised liaison role where health authorities and voluntary organisations are concerned and is known as the HIV-AIDS Liaison Officer. Thus, to some extent, the Community Care Team Leader fulfils at least some of the functions of an HIV-AIDS Coordinator which the authority conspicuously lacks.

Data from the national survey of Social Services and Social Work Departments show that over two-thirds (68 per cent) of the 65 departments surveyed had recruited for specific HIV-AIDS posts in addition to identifying existing members of management as having overall responsibility for policy and service development.

Departments were asked which personnel had overall (lead) responsibility for HIV-AIDS policy development and which personnel had a sectional or area-based HIV-AIDS remit. Ultimately, responsibility for all services lies with the respective Directors of Social Work of Social Services. However authorities had assigned various grades of staff to undertake the lead role in overall policy development. The highest proportion (26 per cent) located policy responsibility at PO level, (a situation found to pertain in three of the five in-depth authorities). The existing duties of these personnel varied and included officers in charge of Mental Health Services, Chronically Sick and Disablement Services and Fieldwork Services. The emerging role of HIV Coordinators was confirmed by the fact that 25 per cent of departments devolved lead responsibility to these posts.

Only two of the 65 departments could not identify someone with overall lead responsibility for HIV-AIDS policy, but a much larger number of departments (43, 66 per cent) stated that no-one held responsibility on a sectional or area basis. From the replies received to this and other questions in the survey, it is implied that sectional or area based responsibility for HIV-AIDS is devolved via a more informal or ad hoc structure; for example, by contact between 'key workers' or informal contact between staff who had received HIV-AIDS training or who had expressed a willingness to act as a departmental contact. Only eight of the 65 departments specified that an individual had been designated formally to undertake HIV-AIDS coordination in each division or area office of the department.

Planning Groups and Working Parties

All five study authorities have Planning Groups and Working Parties, both internal local authority groups and those designed to foster links between the local authority and other organisations. Formal joint-planning mechanisms and arrangements between local authorities and health authorities are excluded from this section.

Hammersmith and Fulham does not have an 'external' group. Planning and information exchange with other organisations takes place via the joint-planning machinery. It does possess an internal group—the AIDS/ARC Policy and Practice Group—on which the Terrence Higgins Trust is present to represent the consumer. According to the HIV-AIDS Coordinator, it has proved 'absolutely invaluable' in the development of policy. Membership includes service managers, field staff and HIV-AIDS specialists from the emerging Unit. Its importance lies in the conscious inclusion of a variety of service managers and field staff.

A superficially similar group, known as the HIV-AIDS Advisory group, exists in Westminster. It has a wide membership including the OT Team Leader (HIV-AIDS), hospital social worker representatives, the Monitoring Officer, the HIV-AIDS Training Officer, a representative from the Personnel Department, the Fostering Adoption Team Leader from the Children and Families Division, the Assistant Divisional Director from the Elderly Domiciliary Care Division, the HIV-AIDS Home Care Team Leader and, finally, the HIV-AIDS Community Care Team Leader plus its Administrator. It is chaired by the Assistant Divisional Director (Disability and Health) who has responsibility for HIV-AIDS issues in the borough. Despite the range of participants, this group does not have the same kind of central importance as the AIDS/ARC Policy and Practice Group in Hammersmith and Fulham. It appears to be essentially an information exchange mechanism. A central weakness in the Group is the absence of field social work staff.

For some time, Kensington and Chelsea had no Departmental planning group. This is perhaps surprising, considering that the HIV-AIDS Coordinator was appointed early. In its absence, the Health Promotion and AIDS Information Officer based in Environmental Health took the lead in establishing an inter-departmental HIV-AIDS liaison group. However, a planning group emerged in the Social Services Department, largely because of the four appointments made out for the 1989–90 grant.

Manchester has a web of internal planning groups comprising the AIDS Working Party, the Equal Opportunities Gay Men's Sub-committee, the Public Education Officer's (men who have sex with men) Support Group and the AIDS in Education Group (MAEG). The AIDS Working Party was originally established at the suggestion of the Gay Men's sub-committee and contains officers from 'frontline' departments as well as counsellors and voluntary organisations. The presence of officers from other departments is further evidence of the authority's corporate approach to HIV-AIDS. The presence of counsellors is also interesting. They are not found on groups in other authorities.

The major 'external' group in Manchester is the Manchester AIDS Forum (MAF). It has emerged out of 'ad hoc' health group established in 1984 at the Manchester Gay Centre. In 1985, a 'medical steering group' was formed with representatives from the three district health authorities in Manchester, voluntary groups, Community Health Councils (CHCs), the local authority, doctors and the Public Health Laboratory service. Since then, membership has grown. MAFs initial emphasis was on health rather than social issues, which is not surprising given its origins and membership. However, this has changed.

Broadly speaking, the main division on MAF is between the health professionals and other, more generalist members. MAF is primarily a practice-oriented liaison body, less interested in 'policy' than in promoting good working relationships and the exchange of information. It is tacitly accepted that organisations and groups represented on MAF will have their own priorities and perspectives but that these can be guided and influenced by committed and informed practitioners. Influencing 'policy' in a 'top down' way is not, therefore, MAF's first priority. MAF's Secretary described its role as:

> '. . . bringing people together to exchange ideas, support each other and *where possible* to influence policy' (emphasis added).

Lothian has developed a cluster of internal planning groups. The AIDS Advisory group was, until recently, the most important. Chaired by the Deputy Director, it met monthly and included 'everyone with HIV-AIDS in their title', ie the HIV-AIDS Coordinator, the three advisors and the HIV-AIDS Training Officer. It now meets quarterly and its membership has been expanded to include two recently appointed drug outreach workers based in Area Offices and a Women's Development Worker. The move to quarterly meetings is part of a deliberate strategy on the part of the Coordinator to broader the focus of AIDS thinking inside the department to include drugs. This has involved the relegation of the AIDS Advisory Group and the creation of two new groups: the Drugs and AIDS Advisory Group and the Drugs and AIDS Practitioners Group.

Membership of the Drugs and AIDS Practitioners Group is open to representatives of voluntary organisations. The Coordinator links the Drugs and AIDS Practitioners Group and the Drugs and AIDS Advisory Group. There are clear parallels between the Drugs and AIDS Practitioners Group and the AIDS/ARC Policy and Practice Group in Hammersmith and Fulham. Both have been deliberately designed to draw on practitioners' experience and to provide them with a channel for raising key practice and service issues.

Lothian has three external planning and coordinating forums. These are the Regional AIDS Group (RAG), the Lothian AIDS Forum (LAF) and, finally, the Joint Planning Team (JPT) Working Party on Addictions. HIV-AIDS has been grafted onto this Working Party. RAG was originally formed as a support/consultative group for the Regional AIDS Coordinator but has since come to be regarded as having a more explicitly proactive corporate role in policy development. It has 14 members including the Assistant Director (Corporate Planning), the Assistant Director (Education), Director (Corporate Planning), the Assistant Director (Education), the Chief Environmental Officer from Edinburgh District Council, a GP representative and the Assistant Chief Constable. Because of its senior membership, RAG has attracted favourable comment from some interviewees who see the Group as concrete evidence of high level commitment to corporate policy making. However, others are less optimistic.

In contrast to RAG, LAF (the Lothian AIDS Forum) is essentially for information exchange among and between practitioners. LAF members are people who work side by side on the ground in Lothian around HIV-AIDS issues. LAF was described as having the 'vices and virtues of a typical self-help group". In other words, it provides members with mutual support but, at the same time, is an arena for conflict and division over and around HIV-AIDS issues. The HIV-AIDS Coordinator sees this as 'a healthy process'.

Lothian Regional Council and Lothian Health Board are coterminous but joint-planning is regarded as vestigial and incapable of 'getting hold of AIDS in a routine kind of way'. The Joint Working Party on Addictions was established in 1986 in an attempt to remedy the perceived deficiencies in

115

joint-planning and it is closely interwoven with RAG and LAF. Originally, it was established for non-HIV-AIDS purposes. Its focus was 'purely drugs—well, intoxicants including drugs and alcohol'. HIV-AIDS issues were grafted on because of the Edinburgh drug dimension. About a quarter of the Joint Working Party on Addictions members are found on RAG and/or LAF. This is a substantial overlap and, clearly, a number of members circulate around the core liaison forums in Lothian.

Planning Groups and Working Parties—The National Survey

Departments have adopted different approaches to intra-departmental liaison on service provision and policy matters depending on factors such as the size of the department and the existence of HIV coordinators. Liaison within departments is achieved either formally through the establishment of working parties or informally via key worker contact or through a combination of the two approaches. A total of 19 departments (29 per cent) stated that they had no formal system of internal liaison. Departmental working parties had been created by 25 departments (38 per cent) and 21 departments (32 per cent) participated in corporate (local authority) liaison groups. Specialist teams of key workers had been created in seven departments (11 per cent) and 11 departments (17 per cent) stated that liaison was achieved on an informal basis only.

Departments were asked whether liaison had been established in respect of shared information on HIV-AIDS, policy formation, and 'case' management. Table 4.1 shows the percentage of departments in contact with other agencies in respect of these issues.

The agencies shown in Table 4.1 are the major providers of health care, education, housing and advice. The agencies listed are examples of external bodies with which SSDs and SWDs may liaise and therefore do not represent the total extent of inter-agency liaison. The focus of this list was the major providers of health care, education and housing advice. However the police, the probation service (England and Wales) and the prison service were also included because of their potential role in respect of drug users.

The percentage of departments liaising with other bodies on case management will depend to a great extent on the prevalence of known HIV-AIDS service users in each locality and the procedures adopted for referral. These findings offer an indication only of the extent of liaison but they suggest areas where collaboration might be explored further.

Table 4.1   **Liaison between SSDs and SWDs and Other Agencies**

	Type of Liaison		
	Shared Information	**Policy Formation**	**Case Management**
Other SSDs/SWDs	51%	15%	9%
District Health Authorities[1]	78%	78%	41%
Regional Health Authorities/ Health Boards	43%	29%	8%
Family Practitioner Committees[1]	29%	17%	3%
General Practitioners	25%	8%	25%
Hospices	14%	3%	3%
Specialist HIV-AIDS clinics or relevant hospital teams	60%	25%	40%
Other local authorities/councils	51%	31%	6%
Local education depts	60%	45%	3%
Environmental health departments	55%	49%	6%
Police	25%	8%	1%
Probation service[1]	26%	7%	7%
Prison service[1]	12%	8%	1%
Local authority housing departments	40%	37%	11%
Housing associations housing trusts etc	22%	12%	5%
Advice centres, eg Citizens Advice Bureaux	20%	5%	8%
DSS Benefit Offices	15%	5%	8%
Voluntary or self help groups	60%	29%	19%
Drugs agencies/teams	65%	43%	26%

[1] figures refer to SSDs in England and Wales only.

Management and Coordination Costs in the Study Localities

The aggregate costs of the management and coordination (MC) component of the Social Care Supply Framework in the five study authorities was £547,200 for 1989/90 and a potential one year cost of £709,700. The variation in MC costs between the authorities was wide with a range of £51,100 to £165,100 actual cost and £52,900 to £223,700 potential one year cost. This is related to differences in the managerial philosophy for HIV-AIDS service and strategy development (Table 4.2).

HIV-AIDS Units

The high relative actual 1989/90 MC costs in Hammersmith and Fulham (£122,000), Manchester (£165,100) and Lothian (£119,900) are associated with the creation of HIV Units in the SSD, City Council and SWD respectively of these authorities. Manchester City council in 1987 was the first of the study authorities to set up an HIV-AIDS Unit based on a corporate model of inter-departmental secondments. Both Hammersmith and Fulham and Lothian have developed units within the social services/work department. The managerial elements of these units consist of six specialist staff (five full time) in Manchester, six in Hammersmith and Fulham (all full time), and four in Lothian (plus administrative support in all three units). The costs of these staff, associated expenses and the office space costs were £150,000, £98,503 and £99,246 for the respective HIV-AIDS Units. There has recently been a movement towards such 'unitisation' in Kensington and Chelsea and Westminster SSDs. However, during 1989/90 managerial staffing in Kensington and Chelsea consisted of three distinct specialist posts (Principal Officer, Service Co-ordinator and Joint Planning Officer), which with associ-ated on-costs and overhead apportionments produced a cost of £88,285. No clear managerial structure exists in Westminster (part of the costs of the HIV Community Care Team Leader and of the Assistant Divisional Director for Disability and Health) hence the low relative cost for management of £33,271).

HIV Co-ordinator

The MC costs for each of the study authorities includes the costs of an HIV Co-ordinator, and in the case of Lothian two such specialists (one employed at regional council level, the other in the SWD). This has the least effect on MC costs in Westminster where the HIV Coordinator role in only part of the job description of the HIV Community Care Team Leader. In all the other authorities this is a specialist senior officer post (albeit unofficially in Manchester).

Other Central Mangement

The day to day involvement of the Deputy Directors of Social Service in the HIV-AIDS service development of Hammersmith and Fulham and Lothian

Table 4.2 **Actual and Potential One Year Costs Management and Coordination 1989/90**

Resource and Component	Ham. & Fulham	Ken. & Chelsea	Westmin.	Manch.	Lothian
1989/90 Actual					
Cost £000's					
Management	98.5	88.3	33.3	150.0	99.3
Non-specialist central					
management	11.6	0	13.8	0.7	6.4
Planning groups	11.9	0.8	4.0	5.8	6.4
Other	—	—	—	8.6	8.0
Total	**122.0**	**89.1**	**51.1**	**165.1**	**119.9**
Potential One year					
Costs					
AIDS Unit management	200.1	124.8	40.1	165.1	103.2
Non-specialist central					
management	11.6	0	8.8	0.7	6.4
Planning groups	11.9	2.5	4.0	6.9	6.8
Other	—	—	—	8.6	8.0
Total	**223.7**	**127.3**	**52.9**	**181.3**	**124.4**

authorities and of the Assistant and Divisional Directors of Disability and Health in Westminster SSD had a positive effect on their respective MC costs. Hammersmith and Fulham also had most general input from other senior managers in the local authority (eg the Directors of Developing Planning, Womens and Ethnic Minorities Departments). Total costs for non-specialist central management inputs were estimated at £11,614, £6,418 and £13,775 for Hammersmith and Fulham, Lothian and Westminster respectively. Manchester City Council Environmental Health Department Director and Medical Officer and the Deputy Director of Social Services constitute a Management Committee for the AIDS Unit (an estimated cost of meetings of £724 in 1989/90). No direct input from other central management was found for Kensington and Chelsea.

HIV-AIDS Planning Groups

There were three types of planning forum that the study authorities were involved in (a) joint working parties with the district health authorities (in

England) or Health Board (in Scotland) and the voluntary sector, (b) inter-
departmental groups and (c) local practitioners groups on which the local
authorities have a representation. The costs associated with individuals'
time and expenses incurred through one to three monthly attendance at
such planning groups were highest for Lothian (total 1989/90 cost estimate
of £6,418), Manchester (total 1989/90 cost estimate of £5,782) and Hammersmith and Fulham (total 1989/90 cost estimate of £11,897). All three types of
planning forum existed in Lothian (ie RAG and LAF joint working parties
the SWDs drugs and AIDS Advisory Group and the Drugs and AIDS Practitioner Group). Two types existed in Hammersmith and Fulham (ie Joint
Planning Team for HIV-AIDS with various sub groups looking at specific
issues and the SSDs HIV Policy and Practices Group) and Manchester (the
local authority AIDS Working Party, a consultation group for the AIDS Unit
Public Education worker and Manchester AIDS Forum for local practitioners). Westminster SSD were also involved in two forms of planning
forum: a JPT for HIV-AIDS and an internal HIV Policy Advisory group.
However this only represented a relatively low cost in 1989/90 (£4031) as
the SSD representation on the JPT consisted of only the Assistant Director
and Assistant Divisional Director for Disability and Health, and there was
very little other planning group activity generated from these two working
groups. Similarly small representation on the Riverside JCC HIV-AIDS
group by Kensington and Chelsea authority staff has resulted in relatively
low cost estimate of £769 for 1989/90. Until recently Kensington and
Chelsea had no structured internal planning group for HIV-AIDS. However
since December 1989 an AIDS Steering Group has been developing an HIV-
AIDS service strategy with additional costs resulting from the large number
of local authority staff involved in the negotiations.

Other Costs

The AIDS liaison officers of Manchester City Council are an integral part of
the corporate model the authority operates for HIV-AIDS services. Although
30 named individuals exist across the local authority departments only a
small proportion are currently actively undertaking an HIV-AIDS liaison
role. The cost this represented in 1989/90 is estimated at £8,593.

Potential One Year Costs

The potential one year costs of MC resources in Westminster (£52,900),
Manchester (£181,300) and Lothian (£124,400) were similar to their actual
1989/90 costs. The far higher one year costs of £223,700 for MC in Hammersmith and Fulham is related to the recruitment of four AIDS Advisors in the

SSDs HIV-AIDS Unit, who started work in January 1990 (with an estimated one year cost of £111,029). Kensington and Chelsea also had a significantly higher one year cost compared to their actual 1989/90 cost (£127,300 compared to £89,100). Much of the difference was due to delays during the 1989/90 planning year in the recruitment of the Joint Planning Officer for HIV and the HIV Services Co-ordinator.

4.2 Training

Along with the production of hygiene guidelines, staff training was an early policy initiative in all the five study authorities. Specialist HIV-AIDS training posts exist in Westminster, Hammersmith and Fulham, Kensington and Chelsea and Lothian. Those in the London authorities were funded initially out of 1989/90 grant. In Manchester, the part-time secondment from the SSD has been providing training since the Unit was established.

In all five study authorities, training included short, information-giving and awareness-raising courses and more detailed presentations for particular groups, although home care staff and social workers predominate. Trainers stressed the magnitude of the task facing them expecially in respect of awareness raising which they perceive as necessary for all staff.

There was a strong element of voluntarism in all five authorities. This has the effect of keeping numbers manageable although many of those most in need of training (ie, with unhelpful and negative attitudes to HIV-AIDS) are not receiving training since they are unlikely to volunteer.

The Training and Staff Development Officer HIV-AIDS in Hammersmith and Fulham estimates that he spends 75 per cent of his time providing training, 10 per cent in staff support, supervision and consultation and 15 per cent in administration and meetings. He has a responsibility for overseeing and providing training across all departments in the authority as well as to voluntary organisations. The training programme draws on not only AIDS Unit staff but also Housing Department staff and feelance consultants. Emphasis is put on training as a prerequisite of an effective service to clients. This is not so clearly the case elsewhere.

Kensington and Chelsea has an HIV-AIDS Training Coordinator. Her job description requires her to co-ordinate an HIV-AIDS Training Programme for the SSD. This currently includes one-day awareness workshops for people with little or no knowledge of HIV infection, AIDS and related issues and a variety of more specialised presentations on HIV and drug use,

HIV and counselling, HIV and mental health, HIV and children, HIV and sexuality and HIV and prejudice. A two-day workshop focusing on issues of death, loss and bereavement in the context of life-threatening illnesses is also available.

Table 4.3 shows the number of courses and participants trained between October 1989 and March 1990 on the basic awareness and more specialised courses.

Table 4.3 **Kensington and Chelsea, Training Courses and Participants**

Type of Course	No. of Courses	Total No. of Course Days	Total No. of Participants
HIV Awareness Courses	5	5	67
HIV Specialised Courses	9	17	96
Totals	**14**	**22**	**163**

The HIV-AIDS Training Coordinator in Kensington and Chelsea believes that whilst service specialisation results in the 'marginalisation of HIV' her role benefits from the high level of specialisation in the borough. It provides a foundation from which to develop initiatives, especially training covering counselling, drug use, mental health, sexuality and bereavement. Nevertheless, whilst there are advantages in being part of a group of specialists, it is 'difficult working under different line management arrangements'.

Systematic training in Westminister began later than in the other in-depth authorities. The borough ran an HIV awareness course once a month between October 1989 and April 1990. The course is currently being run every two months and each session attracts approximately 16 participants. Other more specialised courses are on offer. Topics include substance mis-use, HIV and women and children, networking, working with carers, bereavement and loss and basic communications skills. Another course offers training for trainers.

The basic HIV awareness programme attracted the most varied attendance. Participants included administrative staff, occupational therapists, social workers, residential workers, OT technicians and domiciliary care workers. On other courses, there tends to be a predominance of residential and field social workers. Training sessions have also been attended by local Citizens Advice Bureau staff and members of the National Carers Association.

In Manchester, training has been given high and continuing priority since the establishment of the Unit and is largely provided by the secondee from the SSD. Half her time is spent in the AIDS Unit and one quarter in the SSD providing HIV-AIDS related training. She works closely with two other Unit personnel involved with staff training—the Unit Team Leader and, to a lesser extent, the person seconded from the Education Department. This training team has been supplemented by a recent training appointment to the Unit. The secondment from the Education Department is known as the HIV-AIDS Education Officer and he spends half his time in the AIDS Unit and half in the Education Department where he also undertakes AIDS-related training work.

Trainers in Manchester exphasised the need to develop skills appropriate to a wide range of different groups some of whom (like home helps) are central to HIV-AIDS policy development but who have not previously been the target of any systematic training. Trainers in Manchester try to provide training for home helps in their own local offices, rather than bringing them into City Hall which can be intimidating. The major effort has been put into training home help/home care staff of whom 873 have undertaken a basic, introductory course. However, formal training categories include home helps, first aiders, higher managers, Chief Officers, Council members and foster and adoption officers. They also include categories of education staff.

It is hoped that, eventually, the HIV-AIDS liaison officers will be able to take on some training responsibilities. If this happens, the authority will have, in effect, a cascade approach to HIV-AIDS related training. However, there are some doubts over the level of commitment and interest of some liaison officers and this may be an impediment if the authority chooses to move in this direction.

Training in Lothian began with the appointment of the HIV-AIDS trainer who, together with the AIDS Advisors, constituted a 'Task Force', charged with providing a crash training programme for home helps and foster parents. The early training focus on foster parents is another indication of Lothian's initial preoccupation with child care issues.

Approximately 400 (out of a home care staff of 3,500) had attended information giving/awareness sessions by March 1990. A total of 850 out of 8,000 other staff had also been trained.

HIV-AIDS Coordinators stress that they are constantly being drawn into low level, information-giving sessions. They resent this which they see as a waste of time. In Kensington and Chelsea, the Coordinator had to both organise and either present or participate in a considerable number of training events of different kinds. This situation was the direct result of vacancies in the SSD Training Section although the situation has altered with the appointment of the HIV-AIDS Training Officer in this borough. Other local authorities (and their Coordinators) should consider to what extent they expect or require Coordinators to become involved in training. Substantial opportunity costs are likely to be incurred if this is seen as a major role. Departments had generally failed to develop links with NHS health educators, an obvious source of expertise who could relive the burden on in-house personnel.

The background of HIV-AIDS trainers is important. Whilst they are likely to be trained trainers, they may not have experience of training around sexuality. Of course, not all training requires trainers to constantly address this issue but it is likely to be important for certain groups and it will be necessary to at least raise the subject in many sessions. If trainers feel uncomfortable with the subject, then so will the participants.

Most HIV-AIDS training pivots around consciousness raising, attitude changing and experiential issues. The explicit analogy is with race relations. Both trainers and most professional-grade staff conceive of training in this way. There appears to be very little training around specific management and service delivery issues. At the moment HIV-AIDS Coordinators and HIV-AIDS trainers appear to work in parallel with very little real interaction between the two. However, if specific management and service delivery issues were given greater saliency in training programmes, Coordinators would be able to promote discussion of the kinds of service delivery issues with which they are centrally concerned and use training as a focus for thinking about policy-related issues. They are ideally placed to assess 'needs' of HIV positive clients and help shape appropriate management arrangements and services.

Training strategies are conspicuous by their absence. Lothian is a partial exception in that some systematic ideas for the future have been presented in its SWD Stategy for Drugs and AIDS (May 1989). Manchester has produced preliminary thoughts on objectives but these are essentially 'global' (raise awaresess and counter prejudice). They do not address specific issues or answer specific questions. Manchester has produced an 'HIV and AIDS Public Education Strategy: Goals and Objectives' but no equivalent exists or is planned in respect of internal staff training programmes. Some 'planning' or training takes place since obvious groups are being prioritised in all five authorities. However, prioritisation is only part of a strategy.

Training Costs in the Study Authorities

Staff HIV-AIDS training in the five study authorities represented a total actual cost for 1989/90 of £529, 800 and a potential one year cost of £611, 700. The variation in cost of training between the authorities was not particularly large. Hammersmith and Fulham, Manchester, Kensington and Chelsea and Lothian all demonstrated costs in 1989/90 over £100, 000 (£121, 700, £116, 700, £105, 300 and £104, 600 respectively). Westminster had lowest actual costs in 1989/90 for training at £81, 500 but a much higher potential cost of £114, 300. The costs of staff training in HIV-AIDS issues in each study authority consists of two main elements.

Training Resources: The costs of the training co-ordinator, trainers, materials, room hire and so on.

Staff Attendance: The cost of staff time and expenses from their mainstream activities in order to participate in HIV courses. The costs of these two elements are presented below.

Table 4.4 **Actual and Potential One Year Training Costs, £000s**

Resource Component	Ham. & Ful.	Kens. & Chelsea	West.	Man.	Lothian
1989/90 actual costs					
Training resources	67.7	45.4	41.8	75.2	42.1
Staff att. Days	54.0	59.9	39.7	41.5	62.5
Total	**121.7**	**105.3**	**81.5**	**116.7**	**104.6**
One Year Potential cost:					
Training resources	67.7	66.4	48.0	98.5	42.1
Staff att. Days	54.0	59.9	66.3	42.1	72.7
Total	**121.7**	**126.3**	**114.3**	**140.6**	**114.8**

Each of the study authorities had a specialist HIV-AIDS Training Officer on a senior level grade and budgets for expenditure on trainers, materials, room hire and general expenses. The high relative costs for training resources in Hammersmith and Fulham was related to the existence of this post and budget for the whole of 1989/90. Lothian SWD with a cost of £42, 082 had a full time HIV-AIDS Training Officer but few supporting resources available. Manchester had the highest cost of £75,169. Despite having no full time specialist Training Co-ordinator in the SSD, the corporate approach of the authority has meant that a number of the AIDS Unit staff (mainly the AIDS Unit Team Leader and the AIDS Unit Team Leader and the AIDS Liaison Officer for the SSD) have incurred a major time cost in preparing and implementing the training strategy.

Higher potential one year costs for training compared to actual 1989/90 costs are found for Kensington and Chelsea (£126, 300), Westminster (£114, 300) and Manchester (£140, 600). In each case this relates to the inclusion of the full year costs of the HIV-AIDS Training Co-ordinator. However, the largest part of the additional cost at Westminster is due to inclusion of a full year cost estimate of its new training programme implemented for a six month period during 1989/90. This results in a potential ratio of training resource costs to staff attendance day costs less than one, whilst a greater emphasis on training and implementation costs is now found for Kensington and Chelsea.

Training—The National Survey

A number of questions concerning staff training were included in the national survey of Social Services and Social Work Departments:

- which staff have responsibility for the organisation of HIV-AIDS training?

- who provides HIV-AIDS training?

- what topics have been covered in such training?

- which members have received (or are planned to receive) HIV-AIDS training?

- how, in practice, is training organised for existing staff and new staff?

Only four out of the 65 departments surveyed could not identify someone with lead responsibility for HIV-AIDS training. In 54 per cent of departments, this lead responsibility lay with the Principal Officer for Training, or an equivalent post, or with members of a Training Unit. However, in 34 per cent of departments HIV-AIDS training responsibility had been given to an appointed HIV-AIDS Coordinator or a post having a specific HIV-AIDS remit.

When asked who provided HIV-AIDS training, the majority of departments (59 per cent) stated that they used a variety of trainers, both 'in-house' and from other agencies or organisations, for example, health service and health education personnel, members of voluntary and self-help organisations, professional trainers from HIV-AIDS or other training agencies or professionals with expertise in specific subjects such as counselling, the care of people with terminal illness and so on. Only 19 percent of departments used 'in-house' trainers solely whilst 15 per cent of departments used just the services of external trainers. Only five out of the 65 departments stated that their HIV-AIDS training programmes had been affected by a lack of appropriate trainers.

Table 4.5 shows the emphasis placed on basic training, with training for direct care of people with the virus still in the process of development.

Table 4.5   **Provision of Specific HIV-AIDS Training**

Type of Training	Been Provided	Planned Within 6 Months	Not Available	Not Known
Health and Safety inc. HIV-AIDS	81%	3%	8%	8%
Infection control inc. HIV-AIDS	75%	5%	9%	11%
HIV-AIDS counselling	46%	23%	20%	11%
Factual/medical information on HIV-AIDS	91%	5%	3%	1%
Risk behaviour/ prevention	66%	17%	8%	9%
Care/management of people with HIV-AIDS	54%	19%	19%	8%
Confidentiality	63%	14%	15%	8%
Attitude/awareness training	77%	14%	2%	7%

Departments are at different stages in the training process, either undertaking widespread and comprehensive training programmes, being part-way through basic and specialised training, or only just beginning to consider likely needs. Table 4.6 shows the provision of HIV-AIDS training for different groups of SSD/SWD staff by the percentage of departments having provided, planned or not made available this training.

The figures in Table 4.6 confirm the priority given to home care staff and social workers and reflect the anticipated demand for domiciliary support and counselling services. Despite the widely recognised difficulties encountered by people with the virus in terms of mobility problems and the accessibility of their homes due to illness, physical impairment or debilitating fatigue, the lower priority given to the training of occupational therapists who provide a central role in the assessment of mobility problems, the provision of mobility aids and equipment and the adaptation of homes is surprising.

Table 4.6 **Provision of HIV-AIDS Training for Various Staff Groups**

Staff Group	Trained	Planned	Not Trained	Not Known	Not Applic.
Home help organisers	82%	8%	3%	7%	—
Home helps	80%	9%	5%	6%	—
Hospital social workers	75%	10%	9%	6%	—
Community social workers	77%	9%	8%	6%	—
Social work assistants	43%	14%	22%	14%	7%
Residential home staff	65%	17%	11%	7%	—
Emergency duty team	31%	23%	20%	17%	9%
Occupational therapists	38%	20%	25%	12%	5%
Occupational therapy aides	25%	20%	23%	20%	12%
Adult day centre staff	57%	19%	15%	9%	—
Day nursery/centre	51%	18%	15%	8%	8%
Senior staff	74%	6%	11%	9%	—

Given the changing nature of information on HIV-AIDS and developments and innovations in health and community care, departments were asked whether staff had the opportuntiy to 'update' themselves following basic training. A total of 31 percent of departments stated that they offered some form of regular refresher training with a further three per cent of SSDs and

SWDs keeping staff informed of new developments via area staff meetings, staff bulletins and so forth.

Departments were clearly experiencing some difficulty in addressing this issue in that 17 per cent had yet to develop any plans for the training of the new staff and 15 per cent of departments stated that new staff training was irregular or ad hoc.

The problem of planning in the context of unknown demand for services was mentioned frequently. With regard to training policy and practice, 14 departments (22 per cent) made comments which highlighted the difficulty in motivating staff and allocating resources in areas where demand is perceived to be currently 'low' or unknown, for example:

> '[There is a] lack of interest in staff re. HIV-AIDS issues when under-resourced for their present client demand.'

> 'Major unmet [training] needs. Difficult to motivate staff when to date they have not had to deal with any live cases.'

> 'The major problem is a dearth of cases/referrals.'

One comment in particular encapsulated some of the issues facing a number of departments:

> '. . . in common with other SSDs we have found it more difficult to plan services prior to demand than we would a service where the demand already existed. Confusion arose concerning the level of demand predicted. Figures predicted by epidemiologists two years ago were horrific. Demand at field level proved to be different. There were then dilemmas as to how many field workers, home carers to train and when should one train workers for situations which, on the whole, they might not encounter for some considerable time.'

The emergence of HIV infection and the need to review existing policy and practice has occurred at a time when local authorities and the statutory sector overall is required to develop strategies and services for community care as a whole. HIV-AIDS has presented an opportunity to re-examine services such as counselling, confidentiality, infection control and family support which can be utilised for a study of generic services across the board. The same point can also be made with regard to HIV-AIDS training which affords departments the opportunity to develop staff skills and enhance the expertise available to all client groups in respect of personal support, home care, and confidential and empathetic services.

Developments in HIV-AIDS training have proceeded rapidly over the last few years and trainers now have access to numerous publications and training 'packages' in addition to the availability of training places on vocational and other courses, and attendance at conferences, workshops and so forth. Nevertheless, some departments at an early stage in the planning and training process may be about to 'reinvent the wheel', which given the time and resources required to implement training may be inefficient. It is to be hoped, therefore, that departments are enabled to learn from the often imaginative and innovatory training programmes adopted by other authorities and that the dissemination of training experience is facilitated.

Whilst there is a wide difference in the HIV-AIDS training experience between authorities, strategies produced to date show a strong commitment to training and often ambitious and wide-ranging proposals to develop staff skills and coordinate the contributions to community care from professionals and non-professionals alike. However, a number of departments face practical problems in implementing these plans at the pace required to ensure a generic response to HIV-related demand. There is some complacency in the face of perceived low demand in areas outside major cities and conurbations.

4.3   Prevention and Public Education

Prevention is difficult to disentangle from other aspects of SSD/SWD provision but is defined here as (i) public education campaigns and (ii) other initiatives designed to reduce the spread of HIV infection. The latter includes needle exchange schemes with which most study authorities are associated.

There are no specific prevention initiatives as such in Kensington and Chelsea although the borough produces a range of informational literature and posters which carry an educational message and it has recently established a health education group to develop strategies for HIV related health promotion. There are no central 'prevention appointments' and responsibility for prevention lies loosely with the borough's three HIV Coordinators located in each of Kensington and Chelsea's Area Offices.

In addition to the normal range of public literature, Westminster allocates £100, 000 annually in its Blue Ribbon budget to fund the costs (other than staffing) of drug related initiatives. This initiative is used to promote a 'Say No to Drugs' campaign, youth conferences, competitions, and surveys of prostitution. The Drug Dependency Unit at St Mary's, (where a Westminster

130

hospital social worker is based), provides some needle exchange facilities. As in Kensington and Chelsea, the need for HIV education in schools has been noted but progress is blocked pending the successful transfer of responsibilities from ILEA. Prevention is basically part of the Community Care Team's remit which has an outreach social worker seconded to the Hungerford Drug Project and a drug education and development worker.

Hammersmith and Fulham has a fully centralised AIDS Unit which inludes a number of specific, 'prevention posts'. These are the three HIV-AIDS Advisers for accommodation, women's issues and race equality, all of whom have outreach responsibilities. More explicit importance is accorded to prevention in Hammersmith and Fulham than is the case in Kensington and Chelsea and Westminster. Consideration of HIV-AIDS education in schools has advanced despite the pressures of reorganisation. The HIV-AIDS Coordinator has been involved in a consultation exercise, via the Education Transfer Unit, with both heads and governing bodies on the development of HIV-AIDS educational policy.

Similar education/prevention work is being done in the area of housing. Staff from the AIDS Unit have collaborated with the Special Housing Needs Officer plus other Housing staff in giving a number of presentations to Area Housing Consultative Committees. These are 'umbrella bodies' in each SSD Area which link tenants associations with the Housing Department. These presentations were designed to give tenants information about HIV-AIDS with the aim of preventing harrassment. A number of follow-up sessions have also been given to individual tenants associations. No other Component B local authority has promoted an initiative of this kind.

Hammersmith and Fulham has three needle exchanges in the borough. Each is open one afternoon a week and is attended by a social worker and a community worker from Hammersmith and Fulham. In addition, the local authority is part-funding the adaptation/running of premises. Other costs are borne by health authorities. One major service for drug users in the borough is Barons Court Drug Project which is run by ROMA for people on scripts. The local authority is funding two outreach workers based in ROMA as part of a service agreement and Area 3 Social Work Team is providing regular drop-in sessions as part of its outreach work.

Manchester gives an even higher priority to education/prevention than does Hammersmith and Fulham. The importance given to prevention is emphasised by recent appointments to the central AIDS Unit. These include the (i) Public Education Officer (Young People), (ii) Public Education Officer

(Injecting Drug Users) and (iii) Public Education Officer (men who have sex with men). The job description of the Public Education Officer (Young People) notes that the main purpose of the job is:

'To enable to the Council's HIV and AIDS public education strategy, currently in draft, to be implemented in collaboration with Health Authorities, the Health Education Authority (HEA), with the non-statutory sector, with work particularly targeted on the sexually active and potentially sexually active young people in schools, colleges, the youth service and the unattached and their families'.

The public education strategy referred to in the public Education Officer (Young People) job description lays down general objectives such as increasing awareness and understanding of safer behaviour and healthy living in relation to HIV-AIDS in the population as a whole and amongst specific groups.

Manchester also has established the Manchester AIDS in Education Group (MAEG). The AIDS Unit member seconded from the education Department is Chair of the MAEG. The group is believed by those involved to represent 'a successful example of multi-agency, multi-disciplinary work in the field of HIV-AIDS education'. However, its members identify particular problems. As a large 'sanctioned but not owned' group, it is particularly susceptible to changing political and organisational priorities. In its early stages, it enjoyed strong local political and organisational support for its work because of high national focus on HIV-AIDS.

Like Hammersmith and Fulham and Manchester, Lothian accords specific importance to 'prevention'. The basic objectives of the SWD were first outlined in 1987/88 when they were defined as; to contain reservoir of infection, to provide services to people with HIV-AIDS, to establish an information system, to continue to train all staff and to monitor and evaluate the progress. In 1989-90 the first objective was restated and amplified under the heading 'Prevention'. The department committed itself to preventing the spread of infection through the provision of advice and counselling to clients, particularly adolescents and people with a learning difficulty, together with offering outreach to those vulnerable people not already in contact with helping agencies and also participating in region-wide health education campaigns.

Particular emphasis is placed in Lothian on generic social work as a vehicle for prevention. The SWD HIV-AIDS strategy notes that training should be provided at local level within units to 'enhance team development and (promote) local initiatives towards tackling drug abuse and AIDS issues'. It goes on to observe that all area offices will require extra staff to service the needs of drug users with HIV-AIDS and promote behaviour change including safer sex and safer drug consumption.

Like other study authorities, Lothian provided a range of posters and leaflets in its public offices but its public education initiative consists of the annual 'Take Care' campaign (not to be confused with the resource pack currently in use in residential units). This campaign uses World AIDS Day as a 'launch pad' but it continues afterwards with a series of events and publicity. The annual cost is £70,000 and Lothian SWD contributed £6,000.

Three needle exchange schemes operated in Lothian. The first was set up in Edinburgh after the December 1986 announcement by the Government that experimental exchanges should be set up in different areas and the results evaluated. The initial Edinburgh scheme was only open for a few hours on one afternoon each week. This was found to be insufficient but the scheme was not allowed to expand. A variety of explanations have been offered for this including the presence in Scotland of the common law offence of 'reckless conduct' which, it is suggested, had an inhibiting effect. Other explanations invoke the attitude of the Church and sharply differing opinions within the medical profession about the desirability of needle exchange schemes. There are now two fixed needle exchange sites and a mobile bus financed by Lothian Health Board.

Health Education and Prevention Costs

There was a very wide variation in the costs of such prevention and health education (PE) activity between the study authorities. Acutual PE costs were estimated to be £743,400 in 1989/90 for all five authorities, which represented the second highest cost component (after direct social care services (SC)). Lowest actual PE costs for 1989/90 were found for Hammersmith and Fulham and Westminster at £73,200 and £95,700 respectively. Kensington and Chelsea demonstrated costs of £126,100. There was less variation between the potential one year PE costs of the London study authorities at £128,100, £143,900 and £157,800 for Westminster, Kensington and Chelsea and Hammersmith and Fulham respectively. The highest PE costs were outside of London at Manchester and Lothian with respective costs for 1989/90 of £179,200 and £269,800, (£172,900 and £283,700 potential one year costs). These cost variations were related to differences in the role model for HIV-AIDS services adopted by each of the study authorities. Table 4.7 provides details of the breakdown of PE costs across the four areas of activity.

Table 4.7 **1989/90 Actual and One Year Costs, Health Education and Prevention**

Resource component	Ham. and Ful. £000s	Ken. and Chelsea £000s	West. £000s	Man. £000s	Lothian £000s
1989/90 Actual Costs					
General PE/Campaigns	51.4	22.5	13.6	36.1	8.3
Schools/Youth Work	0.7	4.3	—	88.4	186.4
Environmental Health	—	74.8	5.1	29.4	22.5
Drugs Initiatives	21.1	24.5	77.0	25.3	48.6
Total	**73.2**	**126.1**	**95.7**	**179.2**	**269.8**
One Year Potential Cost:					
General PE/Campaigns	130.3	22.5	13.6	45.8	8.3
Schools/Youth Work	0.7	8.5	—	94.6	186.4
Environmental Health	—	74.8	10.2	—	22.5
Drugs Initiatives	26.8	38.1	104.3	32.5	66.5
Total	**157.8**	**143.9**	**128.1**	**172.9**	**283.7**

4.4 Housing

In the Study Authorities

Housing is not a responsibility of SSD/SWDs although in the four study authorities in England, (Hammersmith and Fulham, Kensington and Chelsea, Westminster and Manchester), responsibility for housing is vested in the same local authority. Nevertheless, it is clear that housing is regarded as a key service for clients who are HIV positive.

Housing departments in all five authorities recognised that harassment of tenants who are HIV positive poses a special problem. Statements and outlines of procedures to be followed are incorporated into directives and guidance notes. Kensington and Chelsea has taken this procedure a step further. A clause has been added to tenancy agreements for council tenants, stating that harassment of a person because of HIV infection is a breach of their tenancy agreement. Hammersmith and Fulham have promoted an educational initiative designed to prevent harassment before it arises. Officers from the Unit and the Special Needs Officer together with other housing staff have collaborated in giving a number of presentations to Area Housing Consultative Committees.

In all authorities, other than Manchester, ARC/AIDS is recognised as a condition conferring medical priority as long as people are currently ill and, hence, 'vulnerable'. This 'policy' which is simply a continuation of existing practices takes no account of the episodic nature of HIV-related illnesses nor does it recognise that unsatisfactory housing may hasten the onset of illness in a 'well' person. If they are young and single they may also be disadvantaged by the housing allocation system since they are unable to accrue the appropriate points. Manchester Housing Department notes that it is unlikely to apply the 'intentionality' clause because it's very difficult to prove. However, the test of a 'local connection' might be applied although people approaching the Department from outside the city are usually offered 'low demand property' if there are 'special circumstances'. The Department does not operate with the standard definitions of the legislation but employs its own categories. Thus, people who are HIV positive are rehoused by the Housing Department under a category known as 'Insecurity A'. This category covers all kinds of serious illness, including such things as heart disease, and a referral from the appropriate source is sufficient to have someone registered as 'Insecurity A'.

Data on numbers of people who are HIV positive receiving a service from housing departments is sketchy. Approximately 60 people have been rehoused by Hammersmith and Fulham, a substantial number in ordinary Council housing. In addition, Notting Hill Housing Trust (NHHT) works with Strutton Housing Association, a specialist association set up to provide housing for people with AIDS. Strutton will be managing ten of NHHT's ordinary self-contained flats. However, Hammersmith and Fulham recognised that a number of people will require a more supportive environment. Two examples of initiatives in the borough are the St Mungo Community Trust which provides a 'family home' and a house run by Hammersmith and Fulham Shared Housing which provides two self-contained flats each for two people to share.

In 1989/90, the Housing Department in Kensington and Chelsea saw about 12 people who were sero-positive and homeless. The majority were single people. These applications amounted to approximately 1.7 per cent of the total 700 applications. Approximately ten applications for transfers had been received mostly from single people but one also from a gay couple.

Kensington and Chelsea has experience of providing temporary and emergency accommodation for people with HIV-AIDS. In early 1990 there were five such people out of a total of 210 households in temporary accommodation constituting approximately 2.4 per cent of the total 'emergency housing' population. There is no special policy concerning the placement of people/families affected by HIV-AIDS: they are normally placed in bed and breakfast accommodation. They may also be placed in Council hostels if there is a suitable hostel vacancy at the time and if it is likely that a permanent housing duty will be owed.

Figures must be treated with some caution. Kensington and Chelsea's Housing Department emphasise that no separate records are kept of clients who are HIV positive. The figures are only known because numbers are small enough to be recalled with some accuracy. However, a portion of HIV positive clients are known with certainty since the Housing Department does provide some 'special' permanent housing for people with HIV infection or ARC/AIDS. The housing department does not have responsibility for home adaptations and home improvements which tenants may require—including those with HIV infection or ARC/AIDS. This is the responsibility of the social services department.

Although housing is not a responsibility of SSDs/SWDs, two of the study authorities have developed accommodation initiatives of their own. In Kensington and Chelsea, an 'adult fostering' scheme has been developed— known as the 'Adult Care Scheme'—which places people who are HIV positive or who have AIDS with families and/or carers. This is, essentially, a statutory equivalent of the St Mungo 'family home'. Approximately £120 per week is paid to the carers/families by the SSD. Carers/families also receive bed and breakfast allowance from Social Security. In Lothian, an SWD accommodation initiative has been developed through its Supported Accommodation Team (AIDS). SATA has four Regional Council properties which it owns and manages and ten other properties available to it through management agreements with housing associations. Each tenancy agreement carries with it a particular 'package of care' specifying the kinds of social care which will be made available to clients. Many tenants do not want the care provided but, in the words of the SATA Coordinator 'we are not an accommodation agency'.

Housing Costs in the Study Authorities

Because of the paucity fo information, the only cost figures available are estimates by housing department managers in Kensington and Chelsea and Manchester of the provision of mainstream council accommodation, temporary bed and breakfast and other forms of accommodation arranges by the local authority for people with HIV infection or AIDS.

136

The dwindling stock of council housing has resulted in relatively low priority for housing for single people with HIV infection. For those people affected by HIV-AIDS who have high priority status (ie, single HIV positive parents or young couples with AIDS who are medically vulnerable) there is often a very limited supply of suitable accomodation such as ground floor flats in 'safe' areas.

Bed and breakfast or hostel accommodation is one option open to the local authority as emergency accommodation for people with HIV or AIDS. However, this is also an expensive method for overcoming housing shortages since the estimated cost of keeping a person in bed and breakfast is £15,000 per year and is, moreover, widely seen as inappropriate for people with HIV infection or AIDS. However, once local residency rights have been established, bed and breakfast accommodation is often the only route available to the housing departments for fulfilling their statutory obligations to provide accommodation for people who would otherwise be homeless.

The costs for HIV-AIDS housing and accommodation include only specific staffing resources and estimated expenditures incurred by providing housing advice for people with HIV or AIDS. The highest estimated costs in the in-depth study authorities is for Kensington and Chelsea borough (£24,900). This covered mainstream staff time in the Homeless Persons, Housing Allocations, Management and Repairs divisions of the Housing Departments. This figure includes the additional costs of a research project investigating the housing needs of residents with HIV or AIDS which was carried out during 1989 by Kensington and Chelsea Housing Department, Manchester City Counil incurred costs of £20,000 in 1989/90 largely from the employment of an HIV-AIDS specialist Accommodation Development Officer appointed in that year. Westminster Housing Department costs for HIV-AIDS related work were incurred through the involvement of generic staff. A nominal cost of £2,600 was estimated for the involvement (quarter time equivalent) for six months during 1989/90 of a housing officer who acted as the Housing Department's lead officer on HIV-AIDS. The Housing Department Special Needs Unit provided the focus for the HIV-AIDS related work of Hammersmith and Fulham. The Special Needs Officer and another HIV-AIDS specialist took the lead role in developing the Housing Department's HIV-AIDS policy, practice and provision. However, insufficient information is available to estimate costs in 1989/90.

The costs of housing department staff involvement in joint HIV-AIDS planning forums involving the SSD/SWD, voluntary organisations and health authorities/boards has been included as part of the 'management and coordination' component of Social Care Supply Framework. In addition, the costs of any support attached to accommodation provision (eg SATA) and the HIV-AIDS accommodation adaptations budget in Manchester have both been incorporated within the 'social care and support' cost component.

4.5   Social Care and Support

Specialist v Generic Services

Special money for the development of HIV-AIDS community care provision was first made available to inner-London SSDs in 1988/89. Special money is a strong inducement for authorities to develop specialised services, not least because accounting is made easier and authorities are required to account for HIV expenditures. Of the English study authorities, Westminster and Kensington and Chelsea have established specialised community care services and posts although Kensington and Chelsea is committed to their eventual reintegration into mainstream generic service provision. Hammersmith and Fulham and Manchester have chosen to develop and enhance generic service provision and, in both authorities, this decision is clearly underpinned by a strong and explicit anti-discriminatory stance which emphasises equal opportunities and equal access to services. However, this kind of commitment can also be used to justify the development of specialised services. This is the case in Kensington and Chelsea where HIV-AIDS workers support the development of specialised services on the grounds that they provide an opportunity to work out appropriate forms of service response and also encourage use by clients who are HIV positive.

However, some caution must be exercised when distinguishing between apparently 'specialised' and 'generic' authorities. Even where the generic approach to service provision is evident, workers involved in HIV-AIDS related work can soon be perceived as HIV-AIDS 'specialists'. There is tension in all five study authorities over the development of specialised services or existence of special money. Scepticism about potential client numbers is widespread. Many workers outside the HIV area understand the argument that services are being developed in order to cope with potential demand but are unconvinced that it will materialise. The phrase 'out of proportion', in relation to HIV-AIDS, was closely linked to the expression of professional concern for the interests of other client groups—especially the elderly and children. Additional resources for HIV-AIDS were seen as misplaced since other areas of service provision needed them more. Opposition to special services and special money for HIV-AIDS was found to be particularly marked amongst home care, meals-on-wheels and elderly day centre staff. A number of social workers felt that HIV-AIDS clients are likely to use services for 'practical advice and very little else' and that people with HIV-AIDS have strong non-statutory and informal networks of their own which are likely to supply most of their needs. Some workers felt that it was a mistake to create special services for what are, in the last analysis, common problems. So hostility to specialised services and/or special money is widespread and springs from:

- scepticism over potential numbers
- concern for existing services
- the belief that social work has only a very limited *vis-a-vis* HIV-AIDS
- and that the problems of clients who are HIV positive are 'common problems'

The existence of 'special money' has been accompanied by accusations of 'empire building', particularly from senior personnel in the SSDs/SWD and in housing, education and environmental health who feel their departments have a key role to play but for which money has not been made available.

Social Care and Support Services Costs—Overview

Social service/work department provision of direct social care and support for people with HIV infection or AIDS and their carers, family and friends represents the largest cost component of the SCSF. The total resource cost for the five study authorities was estimated for 1989/90 at over £2.2 million—just under half of total actual cost of HIV-AIDS service supply included in the SCSF.

The costs of each SSD/SWD's HIV-AIDS social care supply varied according to a number of extrinsic factors and the service planning response of the authorities. Important variables are:

- The amount of different types of social service supplied by the SSD/SWDs. The field service structure of each SSD/SWD available for supply for people with HIV or AIDS. This poses the question of 'what is supplied?'

- The number of people with HIV or AIDS (and carers, family, friends) who are using statutory social services. This raises the issue of who are specific services supplied to and how much is supplied?

- The service strategy adopted. The study authorities differed in the extent to which they made use of HIV specialist resources in supplying social care services. The alternative strategy was to use existing generic resources as and when demand arose. This, therefore, relates to the issue of how services are supplied.

- The availability of Central Government funds earmarked for enhancing the supply of social care of people with HIV or AIDS. From this an assessment can be made of who pays for services supplied.

The issues of what, to whom, how much, in what form and who pays for service supply have important implications for total and average costs of the HIV-AIDS social care provided by the study SSD/SWDs. Aggregate and average costs for different service groups are examined in turn below.

Aggregate Costs for Social Care Service Groups

The HIV-AIDS social care and support costs covered six main areas of service supply by the study SSD/SWDs:

- Hospital based social work
- Community based social work
- Domiciliary care
- Occupational therapy
- Goods and services for people with HIV or AIDS
- Other services, eg meals, residential and day care, fostering and adoption, supporting accommodation/caring landlord/lady schemes, town clerk service and prison social work (in Lothian).

Cost estimates for each of the social service groups are presented in Table 4.8.

Table 4.8   **Aggregate Costs 1989/90 by Service Group, £000s**

Social Care Service Group	Ham. & Fulham	Ken. & Chelsea	West.	Manch.	Lothian	Total
Hospital Social Work	151.5	117.2	127.5	28.0	94.8	519.0
Community Social Work	237.3	16.6	52.6	39.7	80.3	426.3
Domiciliary Social Work	31.4	150.5	164.9	0	48.0	476.3
Occupational Therapy	1.7	40.8	34.4	0	8.1	85.1
Goods and Services	37.4	130.0	5.0	15.0	0	187.4
Other	10.4	186.7	33.1	0.6	309.6	459.1
Total	**469.7**	**641.9**	**417.6**	**83.4**	**540.8**	**2153.0**

HIV specialist resources for social care represented a cost of £1.4 million for the five study authorities in 1989/90, which was 67 per cent of total HIV-AIDS social care costs. The emphasis on HIV Specialisms in Kensington and Chelsea and Westminster produced costs of £517,300 and £374,100 respectively (Table 4.9). In each authority this was over 80 per cent of total actual costs of social care costs for HIV-AIDS. In contrast, just over half of the actual costs of social care supplied by the Hammersmith and Fulham SSD (56 per cent) was associated with HIV specialist resources, at £265,300.

Alternative local authority packages of HIV specialist and generic resources for providing social care for people with HIV or AIDS have different cost implications. Specialist resources represent a relatively high fixed investment in HIV social care provision in the short run. This investment in new specialist resources results in high initial marginal costs, which decline with additional HIV-AIDS service users. The use of specialist resources also leads to cost savings by reducing the need to make use of generic SSD/SWD resources. However, unless the level of specialist resource input equals the

Table 4.9   **Costs of HIV Specialist Resources 1989/90 by Service Group, £000s**

Social Care Service Group	Ham. & Fulham	Ken. & Chelsea	West.	Manch.	Lothian	Total
Hospital Social Work	127.9	97.6	120.6	24.0	89.1	459.2
% of total cost	84	83	95	86	94	88
Community Social Work	100.0	0	52.6	27.0	0	179.7
% of total cost	42	0	100	68	0	42
Domiciliary Care	0	144.7	164.9	0	0	309.7
% of total cost	0	96	100	0	0	65
Occupational Therapy	0	33.2	30.9	0	0	64.0
% of total cost	0	81	90	0	0	75
Goods and Services	37.4	130.0	5.0	15.0	0	187.4
% of total cost	100	100	100	100	0	100
Other	0	111.7	0	0	125.8	237.6
% of total cost	0	60	0	0	41	52
Total	265.3	517.3	374.1	66.0	214.9	1438.0
% of total cost	56	81	90	79	40	67

level of SSD/SWD service demand desired by people with HIV-AIDS the cost outcome will reflect some degree of inefficiency in the use of resources. This is a problem particularly faced by Kensington and Chelsea and Westminster SSDs (and also Manchester to a lesser extent) which have purposely developed a specialist approach to HIV-AIDS social care provision.

Supply of Individual Social Care Services: Service Use and Average Cost

The social care services supplied by the SSD/SWDs are used by a variety of people affected by HIV or AIDS. These service users can be people who are HIV positive with ARC or AIDS, their carers, family and friends, children with or 'at risk' of HIV infection and their parents, and other people not infected but who feel 'at risk' of HIV infection.

Average costs of social care supplied to people affected by HIV or AIDS were based on a number of sets of statistics drawn from the in-depth study of SSD/SWDs:

- Estimates of the average number of HIV-AIDS clients (either individuals or individual units such as a family or parent/child) per week in contact with social care service supplied on an on-going basis, ie caseloads for hospital and community social work, domiciliary care and other continuous supply services. From this average costs per client contact-week were derived for specific HIV specialist and mainstream social care services.

- Estimates of the number of people affected by HIV or AIDS who have received a service from SSD/SWD hospital or community social work, domiciliary care, occupational therapy departments, who have been provided with specific purpose grants, special equipment, travel permits or specific personal services. From this average costs per service use in 1989/90 were derived.

- Estimates of the average number of weeks HIV-AIDS service users were in contact with HIV specialist social work and domiciliary care services in 1989/90. This was derived from the estimates of average weekly caseload and numbers of service users over the course of the year.

- Estimates of the total number of service users with HIV or AIDS who have used specialist and mainstream social care services supplied by the study SSD/SWDs over the course of 1989/90.

142

- Estimates of the total number of people affected by HIV or AIDS who were potential SSD/SWD social care service users. The number of residents in an area with HIV (and unwell) or ARC/AIDS offers HIV managers an indicator of maximum potential service user numbers if all decided to utilise social services at some stage during the year. Generic resources are supplied according to individual demand at any one point in time. The investment in HIV specialist resources require estimates to be made of likely requirements for the services they will provide. Average costs per resident with HIV (unwell) or ARC/AIDS of specialist services provide crude indicators of the unit cost of distributing current aggregate levels of such planned resources amongst total potential service users. In practice as the number of service users increases there will be a point at which additional generic resources or the employment of new specialist resources will be required to maintain acceptable minimum levels of service supply per client. This point is likely to be somewhere between current use levels and the potential number of total service users.

The total number of HIV-AIDS social care service users in 1989/90 for the four English SSDs, shown in Table 4.10, are drawn from estimates each authority was required to make as part of its 1990/91 bid to the DoH for AIDS Support Grant.

To allow for over or under estimates of service user numbers, high and low estimates (20 per cent greater and 20 per cent lower than the 'best estimate') were produced for each authority except Hammersmith and Fulham. Because of greater certainty over service user numbers in this authority, adjustments of only 10 per cent either way were made to the 'best' estimate.

Table 4.10 **Numbers of HIV-AIDS Social Care Service Users 1989/90**

	Best Estimate Nos	**% of Total HIV/ARC/ AIDS**	**Low Estimate** Nos	**High Estimate** Nos
Hamm. and Fulham	279	(47)	251	307
Ken. and Chelsea	400	(45)	320	480
Westminster	350	(64)	280	420
Manchester	45	(34)	36	54
Lothian	320	(30)	256	384
Totals	**1394**	**(44)**	**1143**	**1645**

The number of residents with HIV (unwell) or AIDS in an area, outlined in Table 4.11, were derived from a variety of sources. Estimates were provided as part of the 1990/91 bids for DoH AIDS Support Grant by the four English SSDs.

Table 4.11   **Residents in Each Locality HIV+ (unwell) or AIDS**

Local Authority	Residents who are HIV+ (unwell)	Residents with AIDS
Hamm. and Fulham	380	120
Ken. and Chelsea	675	212
Westminster	410	140
Manchester	116	16
Lothian	1036	50
Total	**2617**	**538**

The proportion of the total number of area residents with HIV infection or AIDS using SSD/SWD social care services provides tentative evidence of variations in service utilisation levels. Overall 44 per cent of HIV-AIDS cases in the five study authorities were estimated to be service users. This may be an over-estimate as it includes a range of types of service users such as family units affected by HIV, carers or children 'at risk' of HIV infection who are not included in the HIV-AIDS prevalence statistics. Although based on estimates of HIV-AIDS prevalence derived by individual authorities from a variety of sources, the proportionate service user level is relatively greater in the three London authorities. This is particularly the case for Westminster (64 per cent). The highly specialist approach they have adopted may assist in efforts at raising awareness amongst potential HIV-AIDS service users of the specialist social care services offered by the SSD.

The level of HIV-AIDS social care cost of the SSD/SWD is related to the numbers of service users in a variety of ways.

- Greater numbers of potential social care service users place greater pressure on ensuring adequate supply. Directing resources to HIV prevention initiatives could have an effect in terms of reducing the numbers of potential service users in the medium to long run.

- Increasing awareness and improved image of SSD/SWD services available for people with HIV, ARC or AIDS through resources directed to outreach work may have a positive short-medium effect on service users.

- Increasing availability and suitability of voluntary sector services for people with HIV, ARC or AIDS may have a negative effect on the numbers of SSD/SWD social care users, depending on whether the two sets of services supplied are substitutionary or complementary. The provision of funds to voluntary organisations to develop social care services for people with HIV-AIDS may enhance these effects.

Total Average Costs

Table 4.12 provides details of the average costs per service user of the HIV-AIDS social care supply.

Table 4.12   **Average Cost of HIV-AIDS Social Care Service Supply 1989/90**

Total 1989/90 Costs	Ham. and Fulham £	Ken. and Chelsea £	West. £	Manch. £	Lothian £	Total £
Best user number estimate	1,684	1,605	1,193	1,853	1,690	1,545
Low user number estimate	1,871	2,006	1,492	2,316	2,113	1,884
High user number estimate	1,530	1,337	994	1,544	1,408	1,309

The 1989/90 average cost calculations in Table 4.12 are produced by dividing the actual costs of specialist resources in that year by the estimated total number of service users and adjusting to an annual cost the weekly estimates of generic social care service use provided on the occupational group questionnaires. To derive annual generic costs it was assumed that the weekly supply of HIV-AIDS related service remained constant. Using the 'best' estimate produced an average cost for the year of £1,545 per service user for the combined HIV-AIDS related social care service supply of the five study SSD/SWDs. Allowing for user number uncertainty produced an estimate of average cost of between £1,309 per service user (high user numbers) and £1,884 per service user (low user numbers).

There is some evidence of a negative relationship between average cost and the use of specialist resources. Westminster demonstrated the largest proportion of HIV-AIDS social care costs on HIV specialist resources below but has lowest average costs per service user. The use of specialist resources in Westminster is extensive and covers all the key service areas of a basic package of social care supply for people with HIV-AIDS in respect of hospital and community social work, domiciliary care and occupational therapy. Such an approach enables a focus for developing awareness of service availability amongst potential HIV-AIDS 'customers'. The costs of such work have been included within the SC cost component. In addition a well coordinated network of specialist social care services can provide a firm basis for designing packages of care to meet the specific needs of individuals with HIV-AIDS. A concentration on providing broad specialist packages of HIV-AIDS social care has the potential for achieving some 'economy of scale' resource savings per service user for a certain level of service supply compared to the mixed specialist-generic supply module of Hammersmith and Fulham and Lothian. The risk is that specialist services will not be highly utilised due, for example, to the poor image of the statutory sector with potential service users, producing high average costs per service user. In Westminster, the specialist service has become well utilised.

Community social work, hospital social work, domiciliary care, occupational therapy and specialist budgets for goods and services represent a standard package of social care service supplied by the study authorities for people with HIV-AIDS. Excluding the 'other costs' category of social care provision such as local initiatives developed to meet specific individual needs in each authority (eg SATA in Lothian, child respite scheme in Kensington and Chelsea), comparison of the basic social care packages of each authority can be made. Table 4.13 presents the 1989/90 year and weekly costs per service user based on the 'best' estimate of HIV-AIDS service user numbers.

The main effect of averaging is a relatively larger reduction in the average costs of social care for Kensington and Chelsea and Lothian. The average cost of £722 for Lothian illustrates the very differing nature of HIV-AIDS social care service provision of the SWD, with more emphasis on provision of supported accommodation services and social care for the 'family' unit and children affected by HIV. The provision of the principal social care services for adults with HIV-AIDS is more prominent in the other study authorities. The costs of such care packages are highest in Hammersmith and Fulham and Manchester SSDs at £1,647 and £1,839 per service user-year respectively.

Table 4.13   **Average Costs of Principal[1] HIV-AIDS Social Care Service Supply 1989/90**

Total 1989/90 Cost of Service User[1]	Hamm. & Fulham	Ken. & Chelsea	West.	Manch.	Lothian	Total
	£	£	£	£	£	£
Best user number estimate	1,647	1,138	1,098	1,839	722	1,216

[1] ie cost of hospital and community social work, domiciliary care, occupational therapy and goods and services.

Potential One Year Costs

The potential one year costs of this supply are presented in Table 4.14.

Table 4.14   **Potential One Year Costs of HIV-AIDS Social Care Supply**

	Hamm. & Fulham	Ken. & Chelsea	West.	Manch.	Lothian	Total
	£000's	£000's	£000's	£000's	£000's	£000's
Hospital social work	172.9	156.5	127.5	28.0	94.8	579.8
Community social work	358.2	16.7	134.9	58.1	80.3	648.2
Domiciliary care	31.4	180.6	224.1	0	48.0	484.0
Occupational therapy	1.7	54.7	83.2	0	8.1	147.8
Goods and services	37.4	130.0	10.0	15.0	0	192.4
Other	10.4	218.7	33.1	0.6	309.7	572.6
Total	612.1	757.1	612.8	101.8	540.8	2584.0

Some of the authorities incurred specialist resource supply costs from part way through the 1989/90 financial year. The potential one year costs of these resources have been included as part of Table 4.14 to demonstrate the full year cost impact of study SSD/SWDs current HIV-AIDS social care supply.

4.6 Monitoring and Evaluation

The Study Authorities

All five study authorities operated normal local authority accounting procedures in respect of HIV-AIDS. Budgets have been created and cost headings identify and record HIV-AIDS expenditure in respect of specialist, HIV-AIDS designated staff, HIV-AIDS supplies and services, administration, capital and so on. Thus, the costs of all aspects of specialised services are recorded as they are for other areas SSD/SWD service provision. However, the monitoring of HIV-AIDS expenditure also requires the identification of costs incurred by non-HIV-AIDS personnel and services. Generic and other specialised personnel and services may have clients who are HIV positive or who have ARC or AIDS and these costs also need to be identified in order to fulfil DoH monitoring/cost requirements. Monitoring of these 'hidden costs' is also needed to establish a comprehensive picture of client numbers and service use. Normal accounting procedures inside SSD/SWDs do not provide for the recording of expenditures of this kind.

In both Kensington and Chelsea and Westminster, monitoring forms have been introduced. In Kensington and Chelsea, the HIV-AIDS Monitoring and Evaluation Officer has introduced a form which is completed for each HIV-AIDS client on a monthly basis by all service providers—HIV-AIDS specialist workers, other specialist workers and generic personnel. The form seeks information on the type of work provided/service supplied and time spent. The introduction of the form in Kensington and Chelsea has met with some resistance. A substantial proportion of staff failed to return the forms, complaining of the extra work involved. Others were anxious about confidentiality for their clients. Opposition to 'extra paper work' and social work concern over confidentiality issues have also surfaced in Westminster. Nevertheless, in both boroughs, the system is being refined and information on service costs and use is slowly emerging. Data requirements in Kensington and Chelsea are greater than those in Westminster insofar as the former authority does not have specialist HIV-AIDS social workers of the kind established in Westminster. Westminster's monitoring task is made easier by the fact that it is the most specialised of the study. The range of specialised services provided means that few generic or specialised workers have clients who are HIV positive or who have ARC or AIDS.

Overall responsibility for monitoring lies with the emergent Unit but day-to-day responsibility is located within 'key managers'. The 'key managers' have been chosen to ensure that, collectively, they have responsibility for all areas of service provision concerning people with ARC, AIDS and HIV infection. Those 'key managers' have been given complete responsibility for producing an identified range of information in relation to each of the services for which they have responsibility. The range of information requirements for each service are such that the information can be collated to provide a perspective on (i) the work of each service outlet (ie an Area Team), (ii) an overall service (ie social work), and (iii) services provided for individual consumers which will assist in constructing care packages or identifying the overlap of different services. Each service has a target representing the expected level of service provision.

The primary responsibility for developing the monitoring system in general and the targets in particular will lie with the newly appointed Monitoring and Evaluation officer but an embryonic system has been in place since June 1989. Since that date, key managers have been filling in their questionnaires providing Hammersmith and Fulham with data on the amount of staff time involved in HIV-AIDS related work and the provision of goods (eg special equipment, telephones) and services (eg holidays). Costings have been calculated for HIV-AIDS staff time in respect of (i) community development work (ii) health education work (iii) running local drop-ins (iv) planning. Costings include not only staff time unit costs but also unit costs of items/services provided and the relevant overhead costs including premises, desk space and management and administration. The general feeling among those responsible for developing the monitoring system in Hammersmith and Fulham is that the early figures probably under-represent staff time on HIV-AIDS by as much as half, since 'key managers' neglect to record time which should be included. The early monitoring exercise has been done manually but the new Monitoring Evaluation Officer will be expected to keep the data on computer.

Eventually, it is intended that the monitoring/costing exercise will be used to distribute funds to service providers. Service providers will be given a special money allocation with the rest being held by the AIDS Unit in a central budget. If monitoring reveals that a manager in a key service area is spending more in staff time or provisions than the original special money allocation allowed for, they will receive 70 per cent of the additional funds needed to cover this cost from the central budget. If a service area does not spend its special money allocation, then resources will be removed and transferred to high cost areas. Hammersmith and Fulham regard certain safeguards as essential. At the moment, the service providers are probably underestimating the amount of time spent on HIV-AIDS related services (especially staff time) but the Co-ordinator and others in Hammersmith and Fulham are concerned that service providers may 'overestimate' HIV-AIDS hours once a link is established between budgets and HIV-AIDS work. The use of targets will help counter this possibility. The Monitoring and Evaluation Officer will have overall responsibility for developing a range of targets for service providers but it has already been decided that two performance indicators must be included to avoid any possibility of 'overestimating'. Firstly, service providers will have a planning ceiling imposed on them which means, in effect, that they will not be allowed to claim an extravagant number of 'HIV-AIDS hours' by setting up working parties or discussion groups whilst not actually providing any service. The planning ceiling has not been finally decided on but it is unlikely that service providers will be allowed to spend more than 40 per cent of their 'HIV-AIDS hours' on planning issues. There will also be 'people targets'. In other words, in order for service providers to receive extra funds from the central budget, they will have to demonstrate that the number of people receiving a service is increasing.

Monitoring procedures in Manchester and Lothian lag behind those being developed in the London boroughs. In Manchester, AIDS Unit costs are recorded under the usual local authority headings as are budgets allocated to the Chief Executive's Department and the Education, Housing and Personnel Departments. However, no costs on these are recorded as no specialised HIV-AIDS services exist in Manchester. All clients who are HIV positive or who have AIDS are seen by generic workers or workers from other specialised services and teams. No monitoring system exists to establish either the costs of goods or services or the numbers of clients using different services. Lothian provides a largely generic service to clients who are HIV positive or who have AIDS. A monitoring form is currently being introduced in an attempt to obtain a full picture of service provision and client numbers. The slowness of this development in Lothian can be directly attributed to the fact that it is not in receipt of 'special money', at least not of the kind received by English authorities participating in the study. Monitoring and evaluation in the English authorities has been developed in response to the DoH requirements attached to 'special money'.

Monitoring and Evaluation Costs

Total costs for HIV-AIDS monitoring and evaluation in the five study authorities represent a small proportion of total Social Care Model costs. This was estimated at £76,700 in total for 1989/90, with the costs for the individual authorities falling into two groups:

a) relatively high costs for the three London authorities of approximately £20,000 to £21,000 per authority (see Table 4.15 in Section 4.7);

b) nominal costs for Manchester and Lothain authorities of £5,000 and £10,000 respectively for 1989/90 (see Table 4.15 in Section 4.7).

In each London authority, personnel in the finance and other supporting departments of the SSDs were estimated to have incurred additional time costs from specific HIV-AIDS related work. This was more evident in Hammersmith and Fulham where the Head of Finance Department had produced a series of unit costs for key staff undertaking HIV-AIDS related provision and a Client Information Officer had a temporary, although major, involvement in the setting up of the computer system for HIV-AIDs monitoring.

Specialist resource and potential one year costs vary among the constituent Component B authorities. Specialist resources amounted to 57 per cent and 41 per cent for the costs of HIV monitoring in Kensington and Chelsea and Hammersmith and Fulham respectively. This relatively high level is due to the employment of specific HIV-AIDS monitoring officers in these two boroughs. Westminster incurred no costs on specialist resources in 1989/90. Tables 4.16 and 4.17 demonstrate the much greater potential one year costs of HIV monitoring and evaluation in Hammersmith and Fulham (£50,800) and the high proportion of this consisting of specialist resources (63 per cent). This is mainly due to the inclusion of the full-year costs of the specialist HIV-AIDS monitoring officer recruited in January 1990. The potential one year costs were also higher than actual 1989/90 costs in the other two London authorities amounting to £25,300 in Kensington and Chelsea and £31,300 in Westminster.

4.7 Costed Patterns of Provision in the Five Localities: Overall Summary

Cost estimation for the Local Authority SCSF service components consisted of two sets of cost calculations:

- Actual costs for the 1989/90 financial year.

- Potential one year costs for resources used during the 1989/90 financial year.

Potential one year costs account for the differential timing of local authority resource inputs during 1989/90 by assuming all costs were incurred from the start of the financial year (ie, 1st April). For example, this includes the full year cost estimated for specialist HIV staffing and other recurring expenditures incurred part way through 1989/90. The actual and potential costs were further disaggregated into specialist and non-specialist resource components.

The aggregate actual costs for the HIV-AIDS related service supply of the five study authorities in 1989/90 are presented in Table 4.15.

Table 4.15   **Aggregate Costs of the Local Authority HIV-AIDS Service 1989–90, £000s**

SCSF Resource Components	Hamm & Fulham	Ken & Chelsea	West.	Manch.	Lothian	Total
MC	122.0	89.1	51.1	165.1	119.9	547.2
T	121.7	105.3	81.5	116.7	104.6	529.7
PE	72.5	126.1	95.7	179.2	269.9	743.4
H	n/a	24.9	2.6	20.2	0	47.7
SC	469.7	641.9	41.8	83.4	540.9	2153.5
ME	20.0	21.2	20.5	5.0	10.0	76.7
Total	**805.9**	**1008.5**	**669.0**	**569.6**	**1045.1**	**4098.1**

The total cost of the SCSF components for the five study authorities was estimated at £4.1 million for 1989/90, with both Kensington and Chelsea and Lothian demonstrating costs of more than £1 million. Lower costs were estimated for the other three authorities at £805,900, £669,000 and £569,600 for Hammersmith and Fulham, Westminster and Manchester respectively.

Within the SCSF the highest costs were demonstrated for the social care and support component. This was a total of nearly £2.2 million for the five study authorities, representing 53 per cent of total costs in 1989/90. In each authority except Manchester social care represented between 52 per cent and 64

152

per cent of total costs. In aggregate SC costs were highest in Lothian (£540,900) and Kensington and Chelsea (£641,900), because of the large number of people with AIDS who are actual or potential users of social care services. The costs of social care supply by Manchester was only £83,400 in 1989/90, representing 15 per cent of total costs. Low numbers of potential service users with HIV or AIDS meant a relatively low priority was currently placed on direct social care provision by Manchester City Council.

The non-London study authorities demonstrated a greater level of cost compared to the London authorities on non-direct social care activities. The cost of the MC, T and PE components amount for £955,400 for Manchester and Lothian (59 per cent of their combined total costs) whilst the costs of these areas of service were only £864,900 for all three of London study authorities (35 per cent of their combined total costs). There is some evidence of trade off in the relationship between social care costs and the costs of management/coordination, staff training and prevention and health education. Compared to the three London authorities the emphasis for HIV-AIDS resource use in Manchester, in particular, and also Lothian has been on developing a wide ranging service structure. In London the priority for resource use has been on the provision of direct social care for people with HIV-AIDS.

The authorities differed in terms of the resource strategy adopted for HIV-AIDS service development. Manchester, Hammersmith and Fulham and Lothian had a mixed specialist-generic philosophy to social care provision for people with HIV, ARC or AIDS. The current philosophy in Kensington and Chelsea and Westminster is to use HIV specialist resources for the supply of social care to people with HIV-AIDS. However, in Kensington and Chelsea this approach is seen by the HIV Coordinator as a prerequisite for the long run integration of HIV-AIDS services with existing mainstream services. This distinction in supply philosophy is demonstrated to a large extent by the actual costs of HIV-AIDS social care supply across the five authorities. Table 4.16 provides details of the actual costs for 1989/90 of specialist resources for each component of the SCSF. It presents these costs as a proportion of the total costs for each component (from Table 4.15).

The highest proportion of total SC costs on HIV specialist inputs is found for the two authorities with a specialist philosophy to HIV-AIDS social care supply. This is 90 per cent and 81 per cent of total SC costs for Westminster SD (£374,100) and Kensington and Chelsea SSD (£517,300) respectively. Less emphasis on the use of HIV specialist resources for the supply of social care is demonstrated by Hammersmith and Fulham SSD, at 56 per cent of total

Table 4.16   **Aggregate Costs of HIV-AIDS Specialist Resources 1989/90**

SCSF Resource Component	Ham. & Fulham 1989/90	Ken. & Chelsea 1989/90	West. 1989/90	Manch. 1989/90	Lothian 1989/90	Total 1989/90
MC £100's	105.1	89.1	37.3	156.6	113.5	501.5
Proportion of total MC costs %	86	100	73	95	95	92
T £000's	67.7	49.0	41.8	75.2	52.2	285.8
Proportion of total T costs %	56	47	51	64	40	54
PE £000's	64.6	64.6	70.6	124.6	147.9	472.3
Proportion of total PE costs %	89	51	74	70	55	64
H £000's	—	0	0	13.6	—	13.6
Proportion of total H costs %	—	0	0	67	—	29
SC £000's	265.3	517.3	374.1	66.0	214.7	1437.4
Proportion of total SC costs %	56	81	90	79	40	67
ME £000's	8.2	12.2	0	5.0	10.0	35.3
Proportion of total ME costs %	41	57	0	100	100	46
Total	**510.9**	**732.1**	**523.8**	**440.9**	**538.2**	**2745.9**
Proportion of total SCSF costs %	**63**	**73**	**78**	**77**	**68**	**67**

SC costs (£265,300) and Lothian SWD, at 40 per cent of total SC costs (£214,700). Despite the generic HIV-AIDS service supply philosophy of Manchester City Council, 79 per cent of the costs of their HIV-AIDS social care costs in 1989/90 was associated with HIV specialist resources. This is related to the low requirement for social care supply by the SSD, resulting in a large proportion of costs incurred on a small amount of HIV specialist resource (£66,000 in 1989/90). If statutory service demand expanded in Manchester a greater use of and total cost of generic social work, domiciliary care and other resources would be expected.

The level of specialist resources in the other components of the SCSF varied between the authorities. A generally high use of HIV specialist resources for the management and coordination component of HIV-AIDS service supply was apparent, representing over 86 per cent of MC costs in four of the study authorities. This was slightly lower in Westminster at 73 per cent of its MC costs. In total 54 per cent of staff training costs consisted of HIV specialist resource inputs (£285,800), although most of the generic element was the cost of mainsteam staff attendance at HIV courses.

A large variation in the level of use of HIV specialist resource use existed for authorities' HIV prevention and health education activities. This use bore no relationship to the specialist-generic social care service supply philosophy of the local authority. Although Hammersmith and Fulham, for example, adopted a generic philosophy to social care supply, 89 per cent of its PE costs consisted of specialist resources. In contrast, Kensington and Chelsea (with a specialist HIV-AIDS social care supply approach) only incurred an estimated 51 per cent of PE costs through the use of specialist resources. Within each authority a range of resource strategies have been created (usually by a combination of planning and chance) for different areas of HIV-AIDS service supply. The H and ME components of the SCSF contain small absolute levels of HIV specialist resources of £13,600 and £35,300 in total. Overall for the five study authorities HIV specialist resources make up 67 per cent of total HIV-AIDS service costs in 1989/90 (£2.7 million, Table 4.16).

The aggregate supply cost pattern changes of the potential one year costs for the study authorities' current (ie, 1989/90) HIV-AIDS related services is considered. Potential one year costs of the SCSF components are presented in Table 4.17.

Overall, the higher potential one year costs were related to three main factors:

- Delays in recruiting managerial and fieldwork staff for HIV-AIDS related posts created at the start of the 1989/90 planning/financial year.

- The English study authorities ensuring that all their DoH AIDS support grant allocation for 1989/90 was spent (partly to guard against cutbacks in the next year's funds due to current year underspending).

- The authorities' further development of their HIV-AIDS service during 1989/90 requiring additional resources.

Table 4.17   **Aggregate Potential One-Year Costs, HIV-AIDS Service Supply 1989/90, £000s**

SCSF Resource Component	Ham. & Fulham	Ken. & Chelsea	West.	Manch.	Lothian	Total
MC	223.7	127.3	52.9	181.3	124.4	709.7
T	121.7	126.3	114.3	140.6	114.7	617.6
PE	157.4	143.9	128.1	202.3	287.7	919.4
H	n/a	24.9	5.2	34.5	0	84.6
SC	612.1	757.1	612.8	101.8	540.8	2624.7
ME	50.8	25.3	31.3	5.0	10.0	122.4
Total	**1165.7**	**1204.7**	**944.6**	**665.5**	**1071.4**	**5052.1**

The greatest difference between actual and potential costs was found for the London authorities. Additional potential one year costs for total HIV-AIDS service supply were £359,800 for Hammersmith and Fulham (producing a total of £1.2 million), £275,600 for Westminster (producing a total of £944,600) and £196,200 for Kensington and Chelsea (producing a total for £1.2 million). Additional potential costs of £95,000 (producing a total of £665,600) were estimated for Manchester.

There was least evidence of additional cost in Lothian with a potential one year cost of £1.08 million, £26,300 more than actual costs in 1989/90. The authorities with a smaller difference in actual and potential costs demonstrated a relative stability in the level of resources directed to HIV-AIDS service planning and supply over the course of the year. For these authorities (Kensington and Chelsea, Manchester, Lothian), most expansion occurs at the start of the financial year with only marginal changes to aggregate service levels until the next wave of development at the start of the following financial year. This is particularly the case for Lothian. Unlike the English authorities Lothian SWD was not reliant on any special grant for HIV-AIDS service development. This seems to have enabled resource planning by Lothian SWD managers. The resulting stability of HIV-AIDS resource levels during 1989/90 has been paralleled by a managerial restructuring of HIV-AIDS service supply by Lothian SWD to give more emphasis to the link between drug related work and HIV prevention initiatives.

All of the additional potential costs for social care in Table 4.17 are associated with HIV specialist resources. Both of the authorities which were adopting a specialist model for social care supply for people with HIV-AIDS had relatively high potential one year costs for the SC component of the SCSF. This was £757,100 for Kensington and Chelsea and £612,800 for Westminster. The inclusion of the full year use of HIV specialist resources for social care in Hammersmith and Fulham resulted in potential SC costs of £612,100, an additional £142,400 compared to actual costs. Most of the additional potential costs for this authority were from the inclusion of the full year cost of key managerial and monitoring staff appointed in January 1990, and associated resources for HIV prevention and health education activities. The outcome in Hammersmith and Fulham is that there is less evidence compared to the other authorities of a trade off between social care supply costs and costs of other areas of HIV-AIDS service supply. However, the overall picture from Table 4.17 is that far higher costs are potentially (as well as actually) incurred from the HIV prevention and education activities of the local authorities in Lothian and Manchester relative to that of the London study authorities. Potential one year costs for PE are estimated at £202,300 for Manchester and £287,700 for Lothian.

The potential one year costs of the HIV specialist resources used in HIV-AIDS service supply by the five study authorities demonstrated a similar pattern to the actual HIV specialist resource costs (Table 4.18) and the proportion of total cost they represented. In total specialist resources were 72 per cent (£3.6 million) of potential one year costs, higher than the equivalent actual costs relationship (Table 4.15 and 4.16).

4.8   The Voluntary Sector

Grants to Voluntary Organisations

Four out of the five study authorities have given significant amounts of money to voluntary organisations to develop initiatives around HIV and AIDS. In the main, funding has been for AIDS-specific organisations. Others, notably drugs agencies, have received grants to develop HIV-AIDS related work. Table 4.19 provides a summary broken down according to the primary area of activity of the voluntary organisations receiving grant in 1989/90.

Westminster did not grant-aid any HIV-AIDS specific organisations in 1988/89. This is because few such organisations were borough-specific and councillors were reluctant to fund voluntary organisations which catered for the residents of other localities as well as Westminster. This is a major policy

Table 4.18   **Aggregate Potential One Year Costs HIV-AIDS Specialist Resources, 1989/90**

Resource Component	Ham. & Fulham	Ken. & Chelsea	West.	Manch.	Lothian	Total
MC £100's	206.8	127.3	44.1	172.7	118.0	668.9
Proportion of total MC costs %	92	100	83	95	95	94
T £000's	67.7	70.0	48.0	98.5	35.9	320.1
Proportion of total T costs %	56	55	42	70	33	52
PE £000's	145.3	78.1	95.7	147.7	165.7	632.6
Proportion of total PE costs %	92	54	75	73	58	69
H £000's	—	24.9	5.2	27.9	—	58.0
Proportion of total H costs %	—	100	100	81	—	90
SC £000's	407.8	632.5	569.3	84.4	214.9	1908.8
Proportion of total SC costs %	67	84	93	83	40	73
ME £000's	37.8	16.2	0	5.0	10.0	63.0
Proportion of total ME costs %	63	64	0	100	100	51
Total £000's	**859.2**	**949.5**	**762.3**	**536.2**	**511.5**	**3651.3**
Proportion of total costs %	**74**	**79**	**81**	**81**	**51**	**72**

issue in Westminster. Indeed, one of the borough's explicit policy objectives is to promote:

> '. . . contact with other local authorities in respect of individual hospital patients who are not residents of Westminster (with the aim of) encouraging these health and local authorities to provide effective help and community services'.

The borough has three major hospitals within its boundaries—the St Mary's, Middlesex and Westminster hospitals. Westminster has, however, like other authorities, been involved in funding prevention initiatives—mainly through the use of its 'Blue Ribbon' money, £100,000 per annum.

Table 4.19   **Grants to Voluntary Organisations by Area of Activity, £000s**

Local Authority	Prevention/ education/ training	Housing/ Accomm.	Social Care/ Suppport	Total
Hamm. and Fulham	43.0	—	307.0	350.0
Ken. and Chelsea	16.0	33.0	170.0	219.0
Westminster	55.0	8.0	—	63.0
Manchester	57.3	25.0	158.1	240.4
Lothian	180.0[1]	479.1[2]	144.1	803.5
Total	**351.3**	**545.1**	**779.2**	**1675.9**

[1] Lothian SWD share with Lothian Health Board the joint capital/revenue funding of a Drugs Crisis Centre

[2] Includes Lothian SWD's share with Lothian Health Board of joint capital/revenue funding of an AIDS Hospice.

The fact that 'special money' is allocated to authorities for *personal* social services has implications for the types of voluntary sector initiatives that can be funded from this source. Within the HIV-AIDS voluntary sector, some are heavily service oriented, for example London Lighthouse. Details of grant allocations in the five study localities thus far show that local authorities have tended to fund organisations with a strong service edge. There is, however, little evidence that grants are being made according to any overall strategy. With the exception of Hammersmith and Fulham, grant aid for HIV-related activities has been described as 'pump priming', with authorities stressing the need to support new organisations and development work.

Accusations were made by some respondents in the voluntary organisations that resources were being allocated without consideration of the relative merits of services provided by organisations making applications. A spokesperson for a hospital-based group in London commented:

'Once could question the allocation of resources when the impression is that those organisations who have a high visibility (resources to spend on PR) come off well, and smaller or less publicity-oriented organisations do not'.

A small AIDS-specific organisation in Greater Manchester observed that although 'we are currently monitoring our expenses and evaluating by making budget choices, we feel our future success with funding lies with raising our profile locally'. These comments highlight the need for local authorities to disseminate straightforward guidelines which outline clearly their priorities for allocating grant aid for AIDS related initiatives.

Grants to AIDS specific organisations in Hammersmith and Fulham differ from those of other study localities in that they are made on a 'service agreement' basis. Service agreements differ from traditional grant aid to voluntary organisations in that funding is tied to specific services, rather than all the services that a particular organisation may provide. Monitoring of services under agreement is given high priority, and includes monitoring of service use/take up. It was initially thought that monitoring of HIV-specific service agreements could be integrated with that of Council services. However, after a year's trial period, it was recognised that this proposal will have to be modified. Difficulties with respect to monitoring arising in this trial period related to the fact that: firstly some organisations service people resident in a number of boroughs; and secondly some services under agreement (for example, providing a drop-in service) do not readily lend themselves to a unitary approach to monitoring service take up.

Voluntary Organisations: Service Development

A major theme running through comments made by AIDS specific organisations relates to the extent of growth and development within this subsection of the voluntary sector. Some talked of the 'proliferation' of groups, and others stressed difficulties encountered through rapid expansion. The growth and development of voluntary sector initiatives around HIV and AIDS have been 'demand-led'. On the other hand, 'special money' grant allocations provided an incentive for these developments.

The potential in London for service duplication and gaps is exacerbated by the fact that whilst informal networks within the voluntary sector are well developed, no London-wide, HIV specific form exists for the exchange of information and experience gained by both statutory and voluntary service providers. This contrasts with Manchester and Lothian, where forums exist (Manchester AIDS Forum and Lothian AIDS Forum respectively) to further liaison and cooperation between 'involved' agencies.

A further issue arising from the rapid development of a number of HIV-specific voluntary organisations relates to the need for clear administrative and organisational structures. The development of these in some cases, has lagged behind rapid service growth to meet clients' needs, causing problems, not least in service coordination.

160

Virtually all the organisations allocated local authority grants in both 1988/89 and 1989/90 were AIDS-specific. This, in some cases, created resentment amongst non-specific organisations who feel that they have an appropriate service to offer, and that this has not been recognised by funders. Encouraging non-AIDS-specific organisations to become more aware of and involved in HIV and AIDS does not preclude the need for specialist organisations providing services solely for people with the virus. However, non-AIDS-specific organisations have skills and knowledge which, although not specifically HIV-related, can be used as a springboard to develop specific services for people affected by HIV and AIDS. There may be some truth in one respondent's claim that:

'we feel a degree of irritation that it seemed Government was willing for the wheel to be re-invented yet again rather than take stock and make use of organisations of known ability and some standing. We already had a basic framework for education/outreach, to graft HIV-AIDS into it would have been no great problem (and indeed has not been apart from the lack of cash)'.

Areas where non-AIDS-specific organisations can and do make significant contributions and where many have considerable expertise include housing provision and advice, advice and information on welfare rights counselling and public education.

Costs of the HIV Specific Voluntary Sector

The voluntary sector provides an important input into the overall HIV-AIDS social care provision. The voluntary sector role in HIV-AIDS related service is part of the SCSF. Each voluntary agency active in HIV service provision incurs costs within some or all of the components of the SCSF. These costs are additional to those incurred by the local authorities but are not necessarily complementary since that depends on the coordination between statutory-voluntary sector supply. In the future the effectiveness of the provider-purchaser relationship developed between the two sets of agencies will determine aggregate costs and resource use efficiency. In the SCSF, voluntary sector costs can be represented by the composite component 'V', covering all the sub-components of the SCSF, ie MC to ME. Because of the difficulty of identifying the use of individual voluntary agency resources no attempt was made to determine separate SCSF component costs for 'V'.

A small scale assessment of the total one year actual costs of HIV specific or related voluntary agencies based in (and around) London (national and local), Manchester and Lothian was undertaken. Costs were calculated for a total for 36 agencies who had either:

- completed a voluntary organisation questionnaire;
- completed a voluntary organisation questionnaire and returned a financial statement (for each agency covering one year between 1987 and 1991);
- provided a financial statement only.

For HIV-specific agencies 100 per cent of their costs are assumed to be HIV-AIDS related. Table 4.20 outlines the number of agencies involved in direct social care and support for people affected by HIV or AIDS, providing AIDS awareness training for other professionals/specialists, involved in HIV prevention/education initiatives or accommodation supply for people with HIV/AIDS. This corresponds to four of the components of the SCSF (SC, T, PE, H).

Table 4.20 **Service Areas of HIV-Specific Voluntary Agencies**

Vol. Org. Service Area	Number of Agencies Providing Service				
	London HIV agencies	Manch.[1] HIV agencies	Lothian HIV Agencies	Lothian HIV Drugs & Related Agencies	All HIV Related Agencies
Social Care and Support (SC)	14	3	6	7	30
HIV Training (T)	9	3[2]	3	4	19
Prevention/Education (PE)	9	2[2]	3	8	22
Housing (H)	5	0	1	0	6
Total	17	3	8	8	36

[1] Includes one voluntary organisation based in Carlisle

[2] Includes one voluntary organisation no longer involved in HIV health education and training initiatives because of the development of specialists in Manchester City Council in these areas.

The costs of the voluntary sector response to HIV-AIDS social care and related services is associated with the structure of the individual agencies involved. The total one year cost of HIV-AIDS service supply estimated for the 36 agencies in the costs analysis consisted of three resource components:

- Staff salaries and on-costs, ie consisted of three resource components;
- Non-staff costs, eg expenditures on materials, supplies, overheads, grants to clients/agencies, staff and volunteers expenses.
- Imputed costs for the supply of services by unpaid volunteers. A rate of £6.38 per hour (based on the hourly rate for an HIV specialist Community Care Worker in Westminster SSDs HIV-AIDS Home Care Team) was used to represent the value of volunteers' services.

Table 4.21 presents the aggregated, range and median costs for direct staff and non-staff expenditures of the voluntary agencies and the estimated costs of volunteers' inputs.

Aggregated one year costs for the 36 voluntary agencies amounted to a minimum range of £6.66 million (low cost estimate) to £7.33 million (high cost estimate). Higher costs (probably a third more) would have been produced if all the agencies had provided information on direct expenditures and regular numbers of volunteers. Over three quarters of the total cost is incurred by the 17 London based agencies, at £5.08 million to £5.63 million. The high cost here is associated with the national focus and hence relatively larger scale of operation of many of the London based HIV agencies. For example, one agency, London Lighthouse, contributes a total of £2.9 million to the London high cost estimate. In practice the total costs of the HIV-AIDS service supply if all HIV specific and non-specific agencies operating within the study localities were included would be much greater than the cost estimate produced in Table 4.21.

The major role of the HIV specific voluntary organisations is clearly demonstrated by these cost figures. The cost of the selection of London based HIV agencies alone exceeds the total actual and potential one year costs estimated for the combined HIV-AIDS service supply of the five study local authorities.

HIV specific voluntary agencies require funds in order to meet the costs of staff salaries and non-staff expenditures including the expenses incurred by volunteers and the costs of their training. Table 4.22 outlines the total income received over one year (between 1987 and 1990) for each agency. This amounted to an estimated £6.88 million (at a median income of £68,400), with £5.59 million of this going to 15 London based agencies.

Table 4.21   **One Year Costs of HIV Specific and Related Voluntary Agencies**

Cost Components	Voluntary Organisations				
	London HIV Agencies	Manch.* HIV Agencies	Lothian HIV Agencies	Lothian Drug Agencies	All HIV Related Agencies
Total no. of agencies[1][2]	17	3	8	8	36
Direct Costs					
No. of agencies	10	2	5	6	23
Staff costs £'s	415.6[3]	4.6	756.6	249.1	1425[3]
Non-staff costs £'s	1481.0[3]	80.2	244.1	103.9	1910[3]
Total direct costs £'s	4541.0	84.8	1001	353.0	5980
Cost range £'s	22.6– 2664.0	4.7– 79.6	26.0– 683.6	9.3– 146.1	4.7– 2664.0
Median cost £'s	134.3	—	112.2	51.8	79.6
Volunteer Costs					
No. of agencies	14	2	6	6	28
Total no. of volunteers	1312	69	168	3	1552
Average no. per agency	94	35	28	0.5	55
High cost est. £'s	1085	74.0	180.1	12.9	1352
Low cost est. £'s	542	37.0	90.0	12.9	681.9
Total Cost[3]					
High cost est. £000's	5626	158.0	1181	365.9	7332
Low cost est. £000's	5083	121.8	1091	365.9	6662

[1] Includes one agency based in Carlisle

[2] Some agencies supplied only information for direct costs or volunteers
Includes agencies for whom only volunteers or direct costs have been calculated, therefore the cost estimates are an underestimation for the 36 agencies in the study.

[3] Excludes London Lighthouse, for which no staff/non-staff cost breakdown was possible.

Table 4.22   **One Year Income of the Voluntary Agencies by Sources**

Source of Income	Voluntary Organisations				
	London HIV Agencies	Manch.[1] HIV Agencies	Lothian HIV Agencies	Lothian Drug Agencies	All HIV Related Agencies
Public Sector[2]					
No. of Agencies	12	2	5	4	23
Amount £000's	3255	60.5	666.6	206.1	4188
Range	10.3–	4.6–	11.9–	33.5–	4.6–
	2116	55.9	520.6	67.4	2116
Median	98.1	—	21.2	52.6	55.9
Fund raising/Donations					
No. of Agencies	11	2	6	3	22
Amount £000's	2054	1.5	138.9	39.4	223.4
Range	2.3–	0.5–	1.6–	1.4–	0.5–
	528.9	1.0	66.0	33.5	528.9
Median	141.6	—	10.3	4.6	33.5
Other					
No. of Agencies	6	1	7	2	16
Amount £000's	276.5	10.7	199.5	34.0	520.7
Range	7.1–	—	1.0–	12.0–	1.0–
	123.0		115.0	22.0	125.0
Median	22.1	—	15.0	—	15.0
Total Income					
No. of agencies	15	2	8	7	32[4]
Amount £000's	5586	12.2	1005	279.5	6883
Range[5]	2.3–	5.4–	1.0–	4.5–	2.3–
	2644	73.1	683.6	68.8	2644
Median	98.1	—	25.6	48.8	68.4

[1] Includes one agency based in Carlisle

[2] Grants by Central Government, local authorities, health authorities/boards

[3] Charities grant, Trust grants and sales of goods and services

[4] Four agencies provided no details of income

[5] Not including one agency recording an income of zero.

The costs of volunteers is based on estimates from the voluntary organisations questionnaire of numbers providing a regular weekly input. A total
of 28 agencies included in the costs analysis provided an estimate of their
regular volunteers. High and low cost estimates have been produced based
on all the volunteers providing an average weekly input of half a day (three
and a half hours) for 48 weeks of the year (high cost estimate) and half the
estimated number of regular volunteers providing the same level of service
(low cost estimate). Where available actual time input has been used to
determine volunteer costs.

There were three main sources of income for the voluntary agencies:

- Grants provided by Central Government (ie DoH, via HEA, Scottish
  Home and Health Department, other Scottish Office sources), local
  authorities (ie London Boroughs, the London Boroughs Grant Scheme,
  Lothian and Strathclyde regional councils), health authorities/boards. In
  many cases grants provided to HIV specific voluntary agencies by local
  and health authorities were derived from budgets funded by DoH
  special money.

- Fund raising initiatives and sundry donations.

- Other sources such as grants provided by charities/trusts, income from
  sales of goods and services.

As Table 4.22 shows, less than half of the income received by voluntary
organisations came from non-public sector sources, ie fundraising, donations, charities and sales.

5 Financing Social Care and Costing Patterns of Use

5.1 Central Government Funding for HIV-AIDS Social Care

Local Authority Funding

This section examines the budgets developed by SSDs, SWDs and other local authority departments in England, Wales and Scotland for HIV-AIDS services in 1988/89 and 1989/90. The development of specific HIV-AIDS budgets over this period has been promoted in England and Wales by Department of Health and Welsh Office grants to SSDs for AIDS related services. Earmarked funds have not been made available by the Scottish Office for SWDs in Scotland. Projections of SWD expenditure on HIV-AIDS in Scotland have been estimated by the Social Work Service Group Working on HIV-AIDS. Partly as a result of this Group's findings, the Scottish Home and Health Department has calculated Grant-aided expenditure requirements for HIV-AIDS for inclusion in revenue support grant allocations.

The budgets created by SSDs and SWDs for HIV-AIDS related services vary in size and content according to the number of potential HIV positive service users, the provision of central Government ring-fenced grant and the overall HIV-AIDS service strategy of the authority. For most authorities, the current demand for statutory social care services by people with the virus is as yet small.

Not all SSD/SWDs who are incurring costs from providing HIV-AIDS related services have developed specific budgets. Unless specific monitoring processes have been set up, expenditures from providing mainstream social care services to people who are HIV positive may remain hidden. Where they exist, budgets usually reflect specific resources allocated to identifiable HIV-AIDS related service initiatives. Ring-fenced Government grant for HIV-AIDS increases the likelihood of a specialist budget being created.

Under the Government's 'Care in the Community' reform proposals, the SSD is expected to operate as the 'gatekeeper' to social care for their residents. The SSDs have responsibility for the assessment of individual needs and for ensuring delivery of appropriate services from statutory or non-statutory agencies. The HIV-AIDS budget created by SSD/SWDs reflect service managers' assessment of specific need for statutory HIV-AIDS service development. In essence, they could provide the basis for the future development of the SSD/SWD as an HIV-AIDS service assessor/manager, purchaser and provider within the framework of the White Paper's 'mixed economy of care' (ie, consisting of a range of statutory and non-statutory services providers).

The availability of ring-fenced grant, and the consequential creation of SSD/SWD budgets for HIV-AIDS services enables assessment of the areas of key resource need for HIV-AIDS related service development that are being identified by the budget holders. To date, resources have been earmarked by SSD/SWD managers for a variety of purposes, such as for the employment of HIV service coordinators, for direct social care provision for people with AIDS or voluntary sector grants. The coverage of the identified HIV-AIDS expenditures of SSD/SWDs reflects the current service strategy managers have adopted for this new area of social service responsibility. The role of central Government grant to SSDs for HIV-AIDS social care and the development by SSD/SWDs of specific budgets are discussed below in the context of the planned reforms to social care provision.

The pattern of central Government funding of HIV-AIDS related social services and initiatives has varied between England, Scotland and Wales. Special funding for local social care and HIV prevention services has been the separate responsibility of the DoH, the Scottish Home and Health Department and the Welsh Office in each country.

In England, the increasing numbers of people with HIV infection or AIDS and the potential increase in demand this was likely to represent for the statutory social services, resulted in the DoH providing ring-fenced grant for those SSDs most affected. Hence, inner London SSDs were invited to bid to the DoH AIDS Unit for a share of £2 million in 1988/1989 to be allocated through the joint finance mechanism. Table 5.1 outlines the final allocation for 1988/89.

A large element of the joint finance grant represented a contribution towards general social service expenditures on HIV-AIDS in the 1988/89 financial year only. However, approximately one-third was allocated as the first part of a three year package of funds for specific SSD projects.

For 1989/90 the DoH introduced a more comprehensive national mechanism for HIV-AIDS social service funding. This again consisted of a ring-fenced grant of £7 million, for which social service departments in England had to bid. In making bids, SSDs had to demonstrate that 30 per cent of their total estimated expenditures on HIV-AIDS services would be drawn from mainstream social service budgets (Circular LAC (1), January 1989).

Table 5.1   **1988/89 Grant Allocation—Inner London**

Authority SSD	Joint Finance Allocation £'s
Hammersmith and Fulham	474,180
Kensington and Chelsea	467,170
Westminster	245,000
Wandsworth	195,000
Lambeth	160,000
Camden	107,000
Southwark	92,500
Lewisham	89,500
Tower Hamlets	60,000
Islington	30,000
Hackney	30,000
Greenwich	27,200

Source: DHSS Press Release 88/134, 26 April 1988

The same basis for funding was applied for the 1990/91 AIDS support grant of £10 million.

The DoH funding for social services in 1988/89 was largely an 'emergency' response to the urgent need to support the inner London SSDs who were facing immediate demands on services by people with AIDS. The package of funding developed for 1989/90 was an attempt at a more structured response supporting HIV-AIDS related social service development in English local authorities. By allocating special resources for service development outside of inner London, the DoH may reduce the flow of people with HIV-AIDS to London, who come to use the well developed medical and social care services located there. In general, the social service departments which received the highest level of support grant were those that produced the most innovative applications.

Use of the grant was restricted to revenue expenditures on personal social service initiatives. No capital ventures were allowed to be financed from this source, although in practice ways round this limitation were found. The maximum grant that an SSD would receive was determined by three categories of funding fixed by the DoH. These were a maximum of £1 million for each authority with greatest concentration of people with, or at risk of,

HIV infection or AIDS (classified as Category A authories); a maximum of £300,000 for other authorities which have, at least, a major treatment centre for people with AIDS (Category B authorities); and a maximum of £14,000 for each SSD making an acceptable bid (Category C authorities). Table 5.2 outlines the total AIDS support grant which was allocated to inner London, outer London, metropolitan and non-metropolitan SSDs within the three funding categories. In total, £6.7 million AIDS support grant was allocated to the English SSDs, a mean average of £65,000 per authority.

The greatest levels of AIDS support grant were allocated to the inner London SSDs, which were all categorised by the DoH as either Category A or B authorities. For 1989/90 five inner-London SSDs (Hammersmith and Fulham, Kensington and Chelsea, Westminster, Lambeth and Camden) received a combined grant of £2.3 million, a mean average of £466,000 per authority. The seven inner London SSDs in Category B received just over £1 million in total at an average of £150,000 per authority. In total £3.4 million was received by the 12 inner-London SSDs (an average £282,000 per authority not including the City of London SSD). This was over £2 million more than was allocated to the 18 outer-London SSDs who applied (at £1.1 million; a mean of £62,000 per authority). Only five outer-London SSDs were designated as Category B authorities, the rest received a Category C classification. The seven Category B outer-London SSDs were allocated on average £190,000 per authority, compared to £150,000 per inner London SSD Category B. This reflects a desire of managers in outer-London SSDs for resources to develop an HIV-AIDS service strategy aimed at both direct social care, public education and the construction of a managerial framework for local services development.

A large variation existed in the amount of AIDS support grant allocated to the metropolitan authorities in 1989/90. Whilst only five metropolitan SSDs qualified for Category B funding status, these had a high level of AIDS support grant ranging from £104,000 (Newcastle SSD) to £300,000 (Manchester SSD).

The total allocation they received was £947,000 (at a mean of £189,000 per authority), compared to £543,000 for the five non-metropolitan SSDs with a Category B classification (at a mean allocation of £109,000 per authority). However, all other metropolitan SSDs (31 in total) only received a Category C rating, with a maximum grant available of £14,000. Hence the overall mean allocation per metropolitan authority was only £37,000. This compared with a mean allocation of £260,000, £62,000 and £25,300 for the inner-London, outer-London and non-metropolitan SSDs respectively.

Table 5.2 **DoH AIDS Support Grant Allocations to Local Authority Social Services Departments by Type of Authority**

	Inner London	Outer London	Metro-politan	Non Metro-politan	Total
Category					
No.	5	0	0	0	5
Total allocation £000s	2,330	—	—	—	2,330
Average allocation £000s	466	—	—	—	466
Category B					
No.	7	5	5	5	22
Total allocation £000s	1,048	952	947	543	3,395
Average allocation £000s	150	190	189	109	154
Category C					
No.	1	13	31	32	77
Total allocation £000s	14	164	372	393	929
Average allocation £000s	14	12	12	12	12
Total No.	**13**	**18**	**36**	**7**	**104**
Total allocation £000s	**3,392**	**1,116**	**1,319**	**936**	**6,763**
Average allocation £000s	260	62	36.6	25.3	65

(1) 2 outer-London authorities did not apply for AIDS support grant.

(2) 2 non-metropolitan authorities did not apply for AIDS support grant.

(3) Includes 3 authorities with a total preliminary allocation of £42,000. Final allocation was undecided.

(4) Includes 6 authorities with a total preliminary allocation of £65,000. Final allocation was undecided.

(5) Includes 2 authorities with a total preliminary allocation of £24,000. Final allocation was undecided.

The AIDS support grant has been comprehensively allocated, so that almost every local authority who applied received a grant. Only four authorities did not apply. However, a total of 76 SSDs (73 per cent of all applications) were designated as Category C authorities and so could only receive a maximum grant of £14,000. This was often used (with their 30 per cent contribution) to fund an HIV co-ordinator post or put towards the cost of staff HIV awareness training.

The Welsh Office allocated a total ring-fenced grant of £38,660 to the eight Welsh SSDs in 1989/90 for HIV-AIDS services. This was evenly distributed subsequent to bids submitted by the SSDs on their plans for the use of the grant (mainly staff training). Unlike the DoH grant to English SSDs there was no requirement for Welsh SSDs to demonstrate 30 per cent minimum expenditures on HIV-AIDS services from mainstream budgets. For 1990/91 the Welsh Office have allocated an HIV-AIDS grant of £80,000 to the SSDs on the same basis as the previous year, so that each authority was expected to receive £10,000.

Unlike Health Authority HIV-AIDS funding, the allocations of central grant to the SSDs in England and Wales took no account of the numbers of people with HIV infection or AIDS resident within each local authority boundary. This is partly because comprehensive and comparable prevalence statistics are not collected on a local authority basis, only by regional health authority areas. A number of local authorities in the frontline of HIV-AIDS service development have set up systems to estimate accurately residents and service users with HIV infection or AIDS. A broad comparison of AIDS support grant allocations per person with AIDS can be attempted for London (inner and outer) SSDs, all other SSDs in England and in Wales (Table 5.3). This is based on AIDS cases reported as of March 1989 to the SU for the four Thames Regional Health Authorities, all other English RHAs and for the Welsh RHA.

Table 5.3   **Grant Allocation Per Person with AIDS**

	1989/90 Total Grant Allocation £000s	People with AIDS (March 1989) No.	Average Grant per Person with AIDS £000s
London	4,494[1]–5,160[2]	786	5,718[1]–6,566[2]
Rest of England	2,255	195	11,564
Wales	38.7	12	3,225
Total	**6,788[1]–7,454[2]**	**993**	**6,836[1]–7,507[2]**

[1] Not including the 3 year joint finance funds.
[2] Including the 3 year joint finance funds.

The inner and outer London boroughs received the largest part of the AIDS support grant in 1989/90. However, the average allocation per resident with AIDS for London residents (786 people) was lower at £5,718–6,566 than that for SSDs outside of London at £11,564 (195 people).

As of March 1989, there were 12 people with AIDS in Wales, so that the HIV-AIDS grant provided by the Welsh Office to SSDs in 1989/90 represented an allocation of only £3,225 per person. The difference in these average allocations relates to a significant element of grant being provided for resources other than direct expenditure on social care for people with AIDS. Initiatives aimed at the prevention of HIV, staff HIV-AIDS training and HIV service management and strategy development require fixed levels of investment resources regardless of the number of people with the virus living in a locality.

In Scotland there has been no special central grant for the development of AIDS related services by SWDs. Instead the Scottish Office in 1989/90 and 1990/91, identified HIV-AIDS as a separate service area in its annual Grant Aided Expenditure (GAE) calculations. This is an assessment method used to determine total levels of expenditure to be supported by Government Revenue Support Grant (Scottish Office Finance Circular 10/89, September 1989). The GAE for HIV-AIDS was based on HIV-AIDS cases reported by each Health Board. In these calculations the SWDs of Lothian, Strathclyde and Tayside were assessed to have greatest resource needs for HIV-AIDS services (assessed at £2.32 million of £2.48 million GAE in 1989/90, and £3.01 million of £3.42 million GAE in 1990/91). Table 5.4 provides details of these GAE calculations. As this money is not a ring-fenced grant for HIV-AIDS, it does not represent additional funding available to the SWDs to expand HIV-AIDS related services. According to Scottish Office officials the GAE calculations for HIV-AIDS are included solely as a means of allocating pre-determined levels of expenditure equitably amongst local authorities.

Table 5.4   **GAE Allocations in Scotland**

Authority-SWD	GAE for HIV-AIDS		GAE for all Social Work 1990/91	HIV-AIDS GAE as a percentage of all social work GAE 1990/91
	1989/90 £000's	1990/91 £000's	£000's	
Lothian	1,166	1,574	77,030	2.0
Strathclyde	708	838	261,907	0.3
Tayside	450	605	42,399	1.4
Rest of Scotland	179	406	151,374	0.3
Total	**2,480**	**3,420**	**532,710**	**0.6**

The method used to estimate GAE takes into account the numbers of people within each local authority area with HIV infection or AIDS. This resulted in Lothian SWD having the largest GAE estimate, representing two per cent of the GAE assessment for all social work services in 1990/91. In comparison, the GAE estimates for Strathclyde and all other SWDs (except Tayside) represented only 0.3 per cent of the total social work GAE estimate for 1990/91.

The Social Work Services Group Working Party on HIV-AIDS produced estimates of predicted SWD expenditures on HIV-AIDS social care, support and staff training in Scotland as a whole. They predicted total resource needs in 1990 of £4.4 million. Based on the crude expenditure estimates they produced (Table 5.5) GAE will not cover predicted resource needs for 1989/90 or 1990/91.

Table 5.5 **Expenditure Estimates for HIV-AIDS Produced by SWSG**

	1988 £000's	1989 £000's	1990 £000's	1991 £000's
Services for HIV+ people	667	879	1,084	1,352
Services for children affected by HIV-AIDS	272.7	523.5	929.3	1,450
AIDS related services for adults	384.3	1051.2	2,287.0	4,179.1
Training	205.0	170.0	120.0	120.0
Total	**1,529.0**	**2,623.7**	**4,435.2**	**7,101.5**

The different approach adopted by central Government to funding local authority HIV-AIDS services either side of the England-Scotland border has raised a number of issues, which are summarised below:

1   Both English and Scottish systems for funding HIV-AIDS community care fail to include Housing, Education and Environmental Health Departments. The Department of Environment, as evidenced by their lack of financial support, does not seem to have acknowledged the message from the service providers that adequate housing is a key element in the provision of effective social care for people with HIV infection or AIDS. In England a number of HIV-AIDS related housing and education initiatives have been funded from the AIDS support grant in SSDs. In Scotland such funds have not been available. This situation militates against effective HIV-AIDS social care planning.

2 Providing earmarked central funds for HIV-AIDS social care and other related initiatives has the advantage of reducing the diversion of these resources to or from other areas of social services need. However, the advantages of special money are offset by a number of specific drawbacks associated with the AIDS Support Grant.

3 It is only guaranteed on a short-term basis (one year for the AIDS Support Grant) which makes long-term planning difficult. In addition, authorities have received very little notice of levels of grant provided for the coming year, which has meant problems in spending the money within a 12 month period (eg, because of the usual delays in recruiting new staff and particular difficulties in attracting skilled personnel for short-term contracts).

4 Capital projects are not 'officially' allowed to be funded from the AIDS support grant. SSDs have very limited capital funds available in mainstream budgets.

5 Tensions have been created within SSDs regarding the treatment of HIV-AIDS as a special case needing special money.

6 The need to provide 30 per cent of HIV-AIDS expenditures from mainstream budgets is likely to result in a diversion of resources from other service areas.

The DoH and Scottish Home and Health Department have, since 1988–89, provided a substantial tranche of earmarked funds to Regional Health Authorities and Health Boards respectively for the medical care of people with AIDS and for local HIV prevention and health education initiatives. Joint planning, in whatever form it takes, between the health service, local authorities and the voluntary sector is particularly important for the efficient development of community based HIV prevention and health education intiatives. However, there still seems to be a large amount of uncertainty amongst many local authorities as to the extent of their financial commitment to such areas. This could be reduced through the use of the joint finance mechanism to co-ordinate health authority and local authority expenditures on community based health education, prevention, and social care initiatives over the medium or longer term. The White Paper on community care is unclear on joint planning arrangements. Further clarification, on the role of Government 'forward planning agreements' between statutory and non-statutory sectors (with a focus on goals, outcomes, contract and funding arrangements) are necessary to determine their feasibility for HIV-AIDS community care initiatives.

Funding of Voluntary Organisations

Statutory funding for HIV-AIDS voluntary organisations is allocated in the main through local authority and regional and district health authority grants. Some money, however, is made available through central government's so-called 'Section 64' funding.

The degree of decentralisation/centralisation of statutory grant giving to voluntary organisations is of particular importance to those organisations with nationwide or regional remits. Grants channelled through local authorities and district health authorities more often than not have a 'locality-specific' clause attached to them (ie the money is allocated for services to people resident in authorities' boundaries). Some larger organisations can qualify for such grants by proving either that a proportion of service users are from a particular locality or that services they offer are available within a particular locality. They can, thus, usually filfil the criteria with respect to eligibility for local authority/district health authority monies. The process of applying for funding to every local authority/district health authority within an organisation's geographical area of provision is, however, costly in terms of time and human and financial resources. Moreover, there are considerable resource implications associated with fulfilling monitoring requirements as these are not standardised across different local authorities and health authorities.

Many organisations have expressed concern as to the uncertain nature of the future of central government funding. Given the resource implications for larger voluntary organisations of having to negotiate with a number of funding bodies within a decentralised system, there is a strong case to be made in favour of retaining at least some element of central funding.

The decentralisation of the grants allocation process is of particular importance in London, where many AIDS-specific organisations provide citywide services. One way of avoiding the costs associated with negotiations with a large number of individual boroughs might be to strengthen the role played by the London Boroughs Grants Unit. Currently, the Unit receives funding from 32 London boroughs and the City of London on a per capita basis. None of these monies are earmarked for any particular service area and the Unit receives no AIDS-specific funding. Despite this, in 1990/91 it provided approximately £350,000 to five major London-wide voluntary organisations. Four of these were AIDS-specific groups and one was doing AIDS-related work. Alternatively, an AIDS specific, London-wide source of funding for voluntary organisations could be considered.

5.2 Local Authority Budgets

National Overview

The creation of specific HIV-AIDS budgets by SSDs and SWDs in England, Wales and Scotland has been related to the availability of special money in England and Wales and to the onset of a second wave of HIV infection away from London and amongst drug users and heterosexuals. HIV infection has become an issue for all local authorities because of uncertainties regarding total numbers and residence of people with the virus, a concern to ensure prevention of spread in each locality and a desire for staff to be trained in HIV-AIDS awareness (especially those who provide direct social care services). In London, SSDs' primary concern for resource use has of necessity been directed to developing and providing direct social care services for the greater numbers of identified people with HIV infection or AIDS.

The extent to which SSD/SWDs have attempted to coordinate a response to HIV-AIDS service needs in their locality and the areas of need they have identified for specific resource allocations were assessed by examining the range of HIV-AIDS budgets created. This involved analysis of the budget and expenditure information provided by SSDs/SWDs participating in the national survey (Component C), and by local authority departments in the in-depth study of five localities. Data was collected to assess:

1   The number of SSD/SWDs with specific HIV-AIDS budgets, and the size of these budgets.

2   The proposed or actual use of resources allocated for HIV-AIDS services.

3   The reliance on special money (in England and Wales) and the availability or other sources of funds.

4   The efforts made by SSD/SWDs to evaluate the cost of the HIV-AIDS service.

Table 5.6 outlines the numbers of inner-London, outer-London, metropolitan, non-metropolitan, Scottish and Welsh authorities in the national survey which had specific HIV-AIDS budgets in 1988/89 and 1989/90 and the resources in these budgets. Table 5.6 demonstrates that whilst only 25 of 61 (41 per cent) SSD/SWDs providing financial information had a specific HIV-AIDS budget for 1988/89, this doubled to 51 out of 62 SSD/SWDs (82 per cent) for 1989/90. All of the inner-London SSDs and most of the outer-London SSDs had created HIV-AIDS budgets in or by 1988/89. The expansion in the number of metropolitan and non-metropolitan authorities with HIV budgets in 1989/90 was promoted by the extension of central Government grant for AIDS related social care.

Table 5.6   **SSD/SWD Budgets for HIV-AIDS 1988/89, 1989/90**

	Inner London	Outer London	Metro-politan	Non-Met.	SSD Wales	SWD Scotland
Total no. of authorities[1]	13	20	36	39	8	12
Authorities in study	7	8	19	23	3	8
No. with HIV-AIDS budget[3]						
(i) 1988/89	6	2	7	4	2	4
(ii) 1989/90	7	3	12	19	1	4
Mean budget 1988/89 £000's	249.0	32.6	32.5	31.0	8.25	40.3
Range 1988/89 £000's	27.2–574.0	53.6	3.4–14.0	5–53	0.5–16	3–132.2
Mean budget 1989/90 £000's	497.0	107	48.7	46.7	31.5	112.8
Range 1989/90 £000's	51.0–1090.0	20–280	17.1–300	10.3–175	—	421

[1] Includes the 5 authorities in the in-depth study (ie, 3 inner-London, 1 metropolitan, 1 Scotland).

[2] No information was received on HIV-AIDs budgets from 1 inner-London SSD for 1989/90 only and 2 outer-London SSDs, 3 metropolitan SSDs, 1 non-metropolitan SSD for both 1988/89 and 1989/90.

The largest HIV-AIDS budgets in both 1988/89 and 1989/90 existed for the inner-London SSDs with a mean budget of £249,000 and £497,000 in each year respectively. In contrast, the HIV-AIDS budgets of the other SSDs in England were much smaller, but had also demonstrably expanded between 1988/89 and 1989/90. This was most noticeable for the outer-London SSDs with a mean budget size of £107,000 per authority in 1989/90, compared to £32,600 in 1988/89. For both metropolitan and non-metropolitan authorities the mean HIV-AIDS budget was over £46,000 per SSD in 1989/90, compared to approximately £31,000 per SSD in 1988/89. These outcomes relate to the characteristics of the SSDs who participated in the survey.

The inner-London authorities had all received DoH HIV-AIDS joint finance for 1988/89. This promoted the development of specific budgets for HIV-AIDS in these authorities. In addition, the five inner-London SSDs who received a Category A classification for DoH AIDS support grant in 1989/90 are all included in Table 5.6, which accounts for the high relative mean budget per SSD for inner-London authorities.

Data on HIV-AIDS budgets was available for only one of the metropolitan SSDs in Category B of the DoH funding classification (Manchester was in the in-depth study, no information was provided by Birmingham, Leeds, Liverpool or Newcastle in the national survey of SSDs/SWDs). This partially accounts for the low relative mean HIV-AIDS budget level per SSD in 1989/90 of between £17,000 and £25,000. Whilst most non-metropolitan authorities in the study had developed small HIV-AIDS budgets of under £20,000 in 1989/90, five SSDs (about 30 per cent of those providing budget information) had specific budgets of over £50,000, the largest being £175,000 in Oxfordshire SSD.

HIV-AIDS budgets had been developed by about half of the Scottish SWDs in the study. Apart from Lothian (with an HIV-AIDS budget of £421,000 in 1989/90) these were of very small magnitude in both 1988/89 and 1989/90 (between £3,000 to £23,000). However, this calculation does not include any data from Strathclyde and Tayside SWD. These were the two localities other than Lothian with greatest numbers of people with HIV infection.

There was very little HIV-AIDS funding provided to the SSD/SWDs from sources other than the DoH joint finance to inner London SSDs and AIDS support grant in England, the Welsh Office grant and mainstream expenditures identified for HIV-AIDS by individual SSDs and SWDs. From the national survey a total of four SSDs in England (Leicestershire, Wiltshire, Bolton, Hillingdon) received funding for HIV-AIDS purposes from other sources (ie, joint finance other than special inner-London AIDS funds and regional Health Authority funds).

Very few budgets included resources for grants to voluntary organisations active in HIV-AIDS work. Some funds may of course be diverted to such agencies from mainstream budgets, but future community care packages for people with HIV-AIDS will require SSD HIV-AIDS budgets to incorporate sufficient explicit resources to purchase voluntary sector services.

Other than in the five in-depth authorities, most SSD/SWDs had made very little attempt in 1988/89 to evaluate the total costs or expenditures of resources diverted to HIV-AIDS related services. This was because most costs were hidden within existing social services and required a specific monitoring programme to be determined. In total, only seven authorities in the national survey stated they had attempted a comprehensive costing of inputs related to HIV-AIDS services. However, 17 SSD/SWDs in the national survey could provide an approximate estimate of actual expenditure on HIV-AIDS services in 1988/89. A better record of monitoring expenditures may become apparent for the 1989/90 year, as a result of the specific HIV-AIDS budgets and requirements for expenditure monitoring connected with the AIDS support grant provision.

HIV-AIDS Budget Development in the Five Study Authorities

The five study local authorities have each developed specific budgets for HIV-AIDS in 1989/90. A substantial proportion of these specific budgets (over half in each English authority) consist of DoH AIDS support grant. Table 5.7 details the budgets, original grant received and total grant received by the end of the financial year. In 1988/89 only Manchester did not have a specific budget for HIV-AIDS, although expenditures on the staffing and associated resources within its AIDS Unit were estimated.

The largest HIV-AIDS budgets in 1988/89 were created by Hammersmith and Fulham and Kensington and Chelsea SSDs. These amounted to £574,000 and £467,000 respectively. The other London authority in the study—Westminster—created an HIV-AIDS budget of £245,000 in 1988/89 (Table 5.7). The size and structure of these budgets were determined entirely by the joint finance provided to inner London SSDs for AIDS related services in that year. Each of the three London SSDs received £210,000 for general expenditure on HIV-AIDS in 1988/89, and variable amounts of funds for a three year period to finance specific initiatives. Three year joint finance of £265,000 and £257,000 per annum was allocated to Hammersmith and Fulham and Kensington and Chelsea SSDs, whilst Westminster received only £35,000 per annum for specific projects. However, although Kensington and Chelsea and Hammersmith and Fulham bids for joint finance had been much larger than the amount they finally received (£519,000 and £1,332,020 respectively), Westminster SSD was allocated the full amount bid for.

The important HIV-AIDS service role of the hospital social worker was recognised by the funding packages of the London SSDs in the in-depth study. In each authority, specialist HIV-AIDS hospital social work posts or teams were created in 1988/89, with the special three year joint finance. The

Table 5.7   **SSD/SWD HIV-AIDS Budgets in the Study Localities, £000s**

uthority	1988/89 Joint Finance Grant [1]	1988/89 Total Budget	1988/89 Actual Exp	1989/90 Central Government Grant [2]	1989/90 Total Budget	Total End of Year Grant 1989/90
ensington & Chelsea SSD	467.1	466.5	351.9	500	899.3	502.7
estminster SSD	245	245	?	420	596.8	538.0
ammer. & Fulham SSD	474	574	600	630	1090	—
anchester	—	—	140	300	528.9	483.1-493.1
othian SWD [3]	(135)	261.3	109.4	(1166)	421	—

* Includes the first year allocation of the three year DoH joint finance for HIV/AIDS.
* Not including the three year DoH joint finance for HIV/AIDS, AIDS support grant only.
) Represents Scottish Office Grant-aided expenditure for HIV/AIDS—not special earmarked Central Government rant.

hospital social work role is on the boundary of hospital and community care. The use of the joint finance mechanism to fund HIV-specific hospital social work initiatives enabled decisions regarding responsibility for their role, costs and funding to be kept separate from all other HIV-AIDS related medical/prevention and social service funding. Table 5.8 demonstrates the specific initiatives funded in the three London authorities in 1988/89. Estimates of actual expenditures for 1988-89 against these budgets were available from Hammersmith and Fulham and Kensington and Chelsea SSDs. Approximately £25,000 had to be found by Hammersmith and Fulham from their mainstream budgets although Kensington and Chelsea SSD's HIV-AIDS budget recorded an underspend of more than £100,000. Most of this was due to problems in recruiting staff for specialist HIV-AIDS posts and delays in starting work once appointed.

The HIV-AIDS related budgets and/or actual expenditures of Lothian and Manchester SSDs were much smaller than those of the London SSDs in 1988/89. The estimated HIV-AIDS expenditure by Manchester City Council of £140,000 covered seconded staff in its corporate AIDS Unit and inputs from Education, Environmental Health and Social Services Departments. Lothian SWD had a budget of £261,000 but recorded actual expenditures of only £109,000. Once again the underspend was related to difficulties and

Table 5.8   **Planned Use of 1988/89 DoH Joint Finance for HIV-AIDS by Hammersmith and Fulham, Kensington and Chelsea and Westminster**

Hammersmith & Fulham SSD	Kensington & Chelsea SSD	Westminster SSD
3 Year project joint finance	3 year project joint finance	3 year project joint finance
Hospital social work team £97,510 pa	Hospital social work team £99,200	Hospital based drugs service social workers £35,100
Community social work* £131,670 pa	2 x AIDS Care Organisers £36,460	
Meals/Domestic items £5,000 pa[1]	Domiciliary care team £106,510	
Urgent needs fund £30,000 pa[2]	Occupational Therapy £15,000	
One year joint finance 1988/89	One year joint finance 1988/89	One year joint finance 1988/89
Domiciliary Care* and Training Officer £210,000	HIV Co-ordinator £19,140	AIDS Liaison Officer £18,438[4]
	Hygiene measures £15,000	Training Officer £18,438
	Other [3] £175,860	Social Workers £52,650[5]
		Domiciliary Care Team £109,560
		Special Equipment £10,000

* Non-specialist resources (except one specialist HIV-AIDS social worker post). All other resources in HIV-AIDS specific.

[1] Originally planned to be a meals budget.

[2] Originally planned to be a budget for residential placements of people with HIV or AIDS.

[3] This was for expenditures as required on voluntary organisation grants, education and training programmes, travel permits, telephone allowances and other special needs/ provisions for people with HIV infection or AIDS.

[4] This post was filled for a 3 month period only in 1988/89.

[5] Three hospital based social workers.

delays in recruiting and appointing specialist HIV-AIDS staff. The fewer numbers of people with AIDS requiring direct social care services, and the lack of special money provided to Manchester and Lothian resulted in a less comprehensive identification of specific resources for HIV-AIDS by these authorities.

The HIV-AIDS budgets of each authority were much larger in 1989/90 because of three related factors:

1   The AIDS Support Grant to SSDs in England and the identification of HIV-AIDS service expenditure requirements by SWDs in Scotland.

2   Increasing numbers of people with HIV infection or AIDS using social services in London and Lothian. In Manchester and Lothian there has been an emphasis on directing resources to education and prevention in an attempt to reduce future numbers of people with HIV-AIDS requiring intensive social care and support.

3   An increased emphasis on monitoring HIV-AIDS expenditures, service needs and service strategy development. The mechanism of using specific budgets assist this process.

The HIV-AIDS budgets of the three London authorities in 1989/90 were £597,000, £899,000 and £1,090,000 for each of Westminster, Kensington and Chelsea and Hammersmith and Fulham SSDs respectively. Lothian had an HIV-AIDS budget of £421,000 and Manchester £529,000 (Table 5.7). The AIDS support grant covered the maximum 70 per cent of the HIV-AIDS budget in Westminster. In Hammersmith and Fulham, Kensington and Chelsea and Manchester over 40 per cent of the total HIV-AIDS budget was accounted for by mainstream SSD budgets. In each case the budgets were approximately double that of 1988/89. The highest cost resource input into the budgets is that of specialist HIV-AIDS staff (managers, fieldworkers, supporting personnel) and on-costs. This is demonstrated in Table 5.9 which details resource cost breakdown in Kensington and Chelsea SSD, Manchester Environmental Health Department and Lothian SWD. The table presents a breakdown of the budget into staffing, supplies and services, voluntary organisation grants, administration, transport expenses and transfer payment components.

The HIV-AIDS budgets of each authority in the in-depth study represents a financial assessment of the funds available and expenditures on specialist service provision. This represents the use of resources newly employed because of HIV-AIDS service needs but may also take account of the need to divert existing mainstream resources to provide an HIV-AIDS related service. For example, Lothian SWDs' HIV-AIDS budget includes resources for the provision of domiciliary care for people with HIV infection or AIDS by the mainstream home helps (although those providing the service will have received training in HIV-AIDS issues).

Table 5.9 **HIV-AIDS Budgets in 1989/90. Resource Cost Breakdown in Kensington and Chelsea, Lothian and Manchester**

	Kensington and Chelsea SSD[1] £'s	Lothian SWD £'s	Manchester £'s
Staffing (gross salary)	477,210	308,267	72,110[4]
Supplies and Services	287,050[3]	3,393	68,000
Voluntary Organisations	n/a	25,344[5]	40,000
Administration and Premises	n/a	67,533	n/a
Transport (eg car allowances)	20,000	17,244	1,500
Transfer Payments[2]	125,00	—	—
Totals	**899,260**	**421,786**	**181,610[6]**

[1] The budget includes central management and administration on-costs, and other overhead costs apportionment.

[2] Capital debt financing.

[3] Includes payments for purchased services, children fostering services, councils fees.

[4] Also includes training and recruitment costs and removal expenses.

[5] Non-HIV-AIDS budgets were used for the bulk of Lothian SWD grants to voluntary organisations for HIV-AIDS related services.

[6] Central management, administration and overhead on-costs not included in this budget.

NB: No details on similar resource breakdown were provided by Hammersmith and Fulham SSD; this level of budget detail was not available for Westminster SSD.

The budgets are not a comprehensive estimate of the total economic cost of each authority's HIV-AIDS related service supply. They reflect an 'accountable' financial cost summary. Table 5.10 provides details of the authorities' estimates of maximum 1989/90 expenditures for the resources

Table 5.10   **1989/90 Maximum/Budgeted Expenditures on HIV-AIDS Services[1]: Social Care Supply Framework Components**

	Kensington & Chelsea £000s	Westminster £000s	Hammersmith & Fulham £000s	Manchester £000s	Lothian £000s
Service management and co-ordination	110.1	18.0	77.7	159.1	83.1
Training	51.0	37.4	56.9	89.6	50.5[4]
Prevention and health education	23.5	41.2	117.4[2]	165.6[3]	115.7
Housing	—	—	—	27.5	6.0
Social care and support	373.7	350.1	590.8	22.5	165.4
Monitoring and evaluation	11.0	17.0	25.5	0-10.0	6.0
Voluntary organisation[5]	196.0	63.0	350.0	192.5-223.5	161.1-901.0[6]
Total	**765.3**	**526.7**	**1218.3**	**656.8-697.8**	**587.8-1327.8**

[1] Budgets include three yearly DoH funded joint finance projects.

[2] Includes £4,000 Health Promotion budget held in the Environmental Health Department.

[3] Expenditures incurred by SSD, Environmental Health, Education, Housing.

[4] Includes £2,000 Training Budget held in Edinburgh District Council Environmental Health Department.

[5] Grants could be used by voluntary agencies for social care, self-help groups or health education/HIV prevention initiatives.

[6] Includes grants for capital projects.

covered by their HIV-AIDS budgets. Disaggregation of the expenditures according to the component of the social care supply model indicates the relative resource priorities each of the frontline authorities have determined for HIV-AIDS service development.

The relatively high level of expenditures on direct AIDS social care for people with HIV infection or AIDS by each authority except Manchester (from £165,000 to £591,000 for the other four authorities) demonstrates the current role of the frontline SSDs/SWDs as key providers of social services. Each authority has incurred expenditures on the provision of grant, either to HIV-AIDS specific organisations or to other agencies involved in HIV-AIDS related work (ie, drug agencies, youth agencies), ranging from £63,000 by Westminster SSD to £901,000 by Lothian SWD (this includes major capital outlays on a new drugs crisis centre and an AIDS hospice). This demonstrates recognition by SSD/SWDs of the important service role independent sector agencies have. As yet there is little evidence of the grant system yielding a 'purchaser-provider' relationship between the SSDs and the voluntary organisation receiving funds. The budgets for grants to voluntary organisations providing HIV-AIDS services only represent a purchasing of services by the SSD if the use of such grants are clearly specified by the SSD and are monitored. However, only Hammersmith and Fulham SSD have instigated a form of contracting system with voluntary organisations (called service agreements by HIV managers) which lay down the objectives and monitoring requirement of the specific HIV-AIDS grants they provide. However, this future role may be developed through the HIV-AIDS managerial and coordination framework set up by each authority.

Manchester City Council may be in the best position for a smooth transition to 'enabling authority' status for HIV-AIDS service development. The relatively low demand from people with HIV-AIDS on social services in Manchester to date has enabled planners there to concentrate on developing a comprehensive management framework, with the aim of coordinating training, social care and HIV prevention initiatives.

The role of the SSD/SWDs in HIV prevention and health education is unclear. Table 5.11 demonstrates that the greatest expenditures in this area have been made by the health authorities/health boards covering the study areas of Glasgow (no details were provided by the three Manchester DHAs). However, Manchester, Lothian SWD and Hammersmith and Fulham SSD have all attempted relatively ambitious community prevention projects. In Manchester and Lothian, a significant part of the expenditures in Table 5.10 for the Prevention and Health Education (PE) component were related to specialist AIDS teams in the Education Department (providing teacher and pupil HIV-AIDS education).

The HIV-AIDS budgets reflect the differing resource procurement strategy for this service area of the in-depth study authorities. The budgets can be grouped according to a number of key features within them:

1   **Specialist resources**   For each authority specialist HIV-AIDS resources have covered staff training, direct social care and related initiatives. For example, Kensington and Chelsea, and Westminster SSDs have set up specialist HIV-AIDS community care teams for the provision of practical and emotional home support for people with HIV infection or AIDS, specialist social work and occupational therapy inputs, and a range of special budgets for 'urgent needs' such as special equipment, travel permits, telephone allowances. This has produced maximum expenditure estimates

of £765,000 and £527,000 against HIV-AIDS budgets for Kensington and Chelsea and Westminster SSD's respectively in 1989/90. These authorities have adopted an almost entirely specialist approach to service development resulting in little use of mainstream non-specialist SSD resources. Therefore, non-budgeted expenditure on HIV-AIDS services is relatively low for these authorities. Employment of specialist resources may enable simpler monitoring of HIV-AIDS expenditures, but represents a high marginal cost for the expansion of HIV-AIDS services compared to the use of non-specialist resources.

2   **Mixed specialist/non-specialist resources**   The HIV-AIDS budgets of Hammersmith and Fulham, Manchester and Lothian are indicative of a specialist non-specialist approach to HIV-AIDS service development. Each authority has (like Kensington and Chelsea and Westminster) set up primarily specialist budgets for management and co-ordinating, monitoring and evaluation, staff training and initiatives revolving around public education and HIV prevention. Each of the budgets of the five study authorities covered an HIV-AIDS training co-ordinator and staff training costs, and a specialist team of managers consisting of an HIV Co-ordinator and supporting 'task-orientated' staff. Thus each authority employed officers with a main role of co-ordinating HIV prevention and health education initiatives and promoting joint planning.

Table 5.11   **DHA/Health Board Expenditure on Health Education and HIV Prevention in the Community**

		(1) Prevention and Health Education £000s	(2) HIV-AIDS Total £000s	(2) as a percentage of (1)
Lothian Health Board	1988/89	587	2,275	26
	1989/90	935	4,644	20
Greater Glasgow Health Board	1988/89	183	1,128	16
	1989/90	308	2,450	13
Parkside DHA	1988/89	427	6,530	7
Riverside DHA	1988/89	342	7,374	5
Bloomsbury DHA	1988/89	512	3,416	15

Kensington and Chelsea, Westminster and Hammersmith and Fulham have specific budgets for employing staff for monitoring and evaluating expenditures on social care and support for people with HIV infection or AIDS. The budgets of Hammersmith and Fulham SSD, Manchester MCC and Lothian SWD include a small number of specialist budgets for key areas of direct social care service provision for people with HIV or AIDS such as HIV-AIDS and drug project workers and homefinder social workers in Lothian, HIV-AIDS specialists in community social work teams, domestic needs and equipment budgets and one hospital social worker post in Manchester. However, much of the direct provision of social care in these authorities was expected to be provided by non-specialist community social workers, domiciliary care workers, occupational therapists and other existing social service staff and budgets. Only hospital social work for HIV-AIDS has been developing using specialist resources. The implication of the non-specialist approach to HIV-AIDS social care is that the total expenditures is likely to be greater than that recorded in Table 5.10 for Manchester (£22,500), Hammersmith and Fulham (£591,000) and Lothian (£165, 000).

3   **Budgets for purchasing social care**   HIV service managers in Hammersmith and Fulham SSD have developed a central HIV-AIDS service budget for buying in social care services from specialist and non-specialist fieldworkers in its own department, other departments in the local authority and from the voluntary and private sectors. The 'purchaser' role has been developed further in this authority than in any of the others in the in-depth study. A system of monitoring expenditures from this budget has been set up by the SSD. The expenditure level of £591,000 in Table 5.10 for social care and support by Hammersmith and Fulham SSD represents all expenditures on staff time, other direct service provision and managerial/administrative overheads accounted for by the monitoring system.

Kensington and Chelsea SSD developed a special budget of £30,000 in 1989/90 for purchasing services such as massage and art therapy for people with HIV infection or AIDS but as yet have not set up budgets for purchasing more fundamental social services such as home care. The model constructed in Hammersmith and Fulham is very much in line with Government thinking regarding the implementation of its White Paper reforms for community care, and this therefore received the appropriate encouragement and financial support from the DoH. It is viewed by central and local government as a test-case for the practical application of such service packages in other more traditional areas of social services provision such as that for elderly people.

4   **Local authority resources** The relatively low pressure on social service resource needs for HIV-AIDS in Manchester has enabled the City Council to adopt a corporate approach to HIV-AIDS service development involving all the frontline service departments of the local authority such as the SSD, Environmental Health, Education and Housing. The HIV-AIDS budget involves a series of recharges to the SSD by other local authority departments incurring HIV-AIDS related expenditures. This has produced a maximum expected expenditure of £698,000 (Table 5.10).

5.3   Special Money and Budgets for a Special Service

A number of apparent and potential problems arise from the specialisation of local authority HIV-AIDS services created by the DoH ring-fenced AIDS support grant, the Welsh Office funding for AIDS related services provided to the eight local authorities in Wales and the creation of special budgets (as has occurred in all of the in-depth study authorities).

One danger of special money is that if it is withdrawn then specialist budgets for HIV-AIDS services in the high profile authorities may have to also be reduced. This is of greatest worry for those authorities running a largely specialist HIV/AIDS service which is not well integrated into existing department budget systems (ie, Kensington and Chelsea SSD and Westminster SSD in particular). HIV-AIDS budgets in these authorities exist purely because of the availability of special money.

The expenditure estimates discussed above only represent the direct costs of service provision for each authority against specific HIV-AIDS budgets. They do not include all hidden costs such as the time of non-specialist/non-budget staff on HIV-AIDS work or the costs of central management, administration and other overheads (except for attempts by Hammersmith and Fulham SSD to account for such elements as part of its HIV-AIDS service monitoring) or the cost of staff time on attending HIV-AIDS training courses.

Some disquiet in all five study localities over the development of specialised budgets and special money is evident. Scepticism about potential client numbers is, if not widespread, at least not uncommon. The phrase 'out of proportion' appeared on a number of questionnaires from social workers. A surprisingly high proportion of such comments came from social workers in the three London authorities. In most of the cases, this kind of opinion was closely linked to the expression of professional concern for the interests of particular client groups, especially the elderly and children. Resources for HIV-AIDS were widely seen as misplaced since other areas of service provision (ie, their own) were said to need them more. Hostility to special budgets and special money for HIV-AIDS is particularly marked amongst home care, meals-on-wheels and elderly day centre staff. Even though special money and special services have been made available there is a feeling that services for the elderly are in some way diminished. This sentiment is especially marked in those localities where no specific home care budgets have been developed (Lothian, Manchester and Hammersmith and Fulham). As one respondent said:

'No-one can tell me that my elderly are not going to suffer'.

Some workers are sceptical about the development of special budgets and the need for special money, not because potential client numbers are low or because of their impact on existing services and existing client groups, but because it is said that social workers have only a limited role where HIV-AIDS is concernced. A number of workers felt that HIV-AIDS clients are, in the main, likely to use the services for, as one put it 'practical advice and very little else'. These workers believed that people who are HIV positive or have ARC/AIDS have strong non-statutory and informal networks of their own which are likely to supply most of their needs. Other workers felt that it is a mistake to create special services for what are, in the last analysis, common problems. While some are clearly relieved that specialised services exist to take on what would otherwise be additional work for existing staff, others complain that the creation of specialised services and posts mean that most staff are, in effect, excluded from HIV-AIDS issues. As one respondent in Westminster observed '. . . it's a mistake to create HIV-AIDS ghettoes'.

The existence of special money and the associated development of HIV-AIDS budgets (for specialist services) is accompanied by some accusations of 'empire-building'. However, there is an interesting tension between accusations of empire-building on the one hand and the obvious lack of liaison between workers who could be part of the same 'empire' on the other. The accusation of 'empire-building' is mostly directed at AIDS specialists by other managers who do not have the same kind of deep personal commitment but who feel excluded from the organisational opportunities presented by HIV-AIDS. Special money and special budgets thus appear to create tensions between AIDS workers who have particular expertise and interest and are constantly lobbying for resources and others with less zeal who can see an opportunity for promoting their managerial interests and enlarging their niche within the organisation.

5.4   Costing the Components of Care

The costs of packages of social care and support services used by the respondents in the study were incurred by five main sets of agencies:

- the voluntary sector
- the local authority SSD/SWD
- specific staff employed by the NHS
- the private sector
- informal carers

The services supplied by each agency consisted of a combination of practical and emotional support. Practical support consists of both specific advice (eg financial, diet, sexual) and the provision of goods and services such as mobility devices, bus passes, massage, autogenic training.

The survey demonstrated the use of a number of inter-related types of care/support package by people who were HIV positive or who had AIDS. Five packages were identified for the purpose of the costing of respondent service use:

- SSD/SWD social worker services
- home support services
- practical goods and services
- health maintenance therapy/treatment
- practical advice and emotional support services

Each of these packages represents a key element in an integrated package of social care for people with HIV infection or AIDS. Depending on their needs and the appropriateness of the services provided, each respondent used parts of, all, some or none of these packages.

Method of Assessing Costs

The estimation of the costs of service use was based on the opportunity cost of staff, volunteers and informal carer time inputs, equipment provided and facilities used (this is the cost of not using resources in an alternative service). The costs of service use did not include an estimate of the expenses of time and money incurred by respondents in using a service. The only personal cost of HIV related service use that were included were the estimated expenditures on the purchase of private services.

The calculation of the average costs of service use involved a number of methods:

Firstly, average weekly costs of service use by respondent and individual service user were calculated. The costs of services used less frequently than once per week were converted to an average weekly cost. Where respondents had stated they used services on a number of occasions only (eg, three or four times) or on a one-off basis (eg, such as house moving services, occupational therapist), the weekly cost was based on this service use occurring over the course of the past year (ie, total cost divided by 52 weeks). Therefore, the weekly costs represents a maximum potential amount over a year of service use.

Secondly, a high and a low estimate of weekly service use was determined for each of the packages of social care/support. The basis for these cost estimates varied for each package, and are outlined in detail within the discussion of the costs of individual packages below. In a number of instances it was not known whether a service was supplied by an HIV-AIDS specialist worker or a volunteer or a non-specialist. For social worker, and statutory and voluntary sector supplied home support and practical services a high cost estimate included an assumption that the service was supplied by a specialist worker/volunteer. The low cost estimate included the assumption that service supply was by non-specialists whose services for people with HIV infection or AIDS were valued slightly below that of HIV-AIDS specialists.

In addition, the unit costs of non-specialists incorporated lower apportionment of overhead and central establishment costs and local management and administrative support costs. This was based on the assumption that less of these resources were diverted to HIV-AIDS related service supply for non-specialists compared to specialist service provision. For some HIV-AIDS voluntary agency services the high cost estimate incorporated the assumption that service supply was by a paid worker whilst the low cost estimate was based on service supply by a trained volunteer. Other unit cost variations were based on different estimates of level of service use. For example, the high and low cost estimates of the use of telephone helpline services were based on telephone calls of an average of 30 minutes and 10 minutes respectively.

The costs of statutory and voluntary agency paid staff time used by respondents were higher in London than in Manchester, Scotland and Birmingham because of the inclusion of London weighting in salaries.

Weekly Costs per Respondent of Service Packages

For all respondents (n = 181), the weekly cost estimated for social care and support service use was £45.12 per respondent based on a high cost estimate. The low cost estimate was £37.14 per respondent (Table 5.12).

Table 5.12   **Average Weekly Costs per Respondent of Five Packages of Social Care/ Support by HIV Status**

Type of Social Care	Weekly Costs (£ per week)			
	HIV+ (n=106)	ARC (n=35)	AIDS (n=40)	Total (n=181)
Home Support				
low cost estimate	10.35	26.07	70.45	26.67
high cost estimate	10.87	32.74	82.78	30.99
Social Worker				
low cost estimate	2.47	4.77	5.83	3.52
high cost estimate	3.17	6.31	7.97	5.28
Practical Goods and Services				
low cost estimate	2.76	7.02	8.51	4.85
high cost estimate	2.76	7.02	8.59	4.87
Health Maintenance Therapy/Treatment				
low cost estimate	1.41	1.11	2.75	1.64
high cost estimate	2.14	4.40	5.94	3.41
Practical and Emotional Support Services				
low cost estimate	0.42	0.57	0.56	0.46
high cost estimate	0.54	0.66	0.56	0.57
Total Integrated Package				
low cost estimate	17.41	39.53	88.11	37.14
high cost estimate	19.48	51.13	105.84	45.12

Variations between the average costs of the service use packages existed. The highest weekly cost was found for home support services at £30.99 (high cost estimate) or £26.67) (low cost estimate). This consisted of the use of SSD/SWD domiciliary care, voluntary care, voluntary agency home support services such as buddies and practical help in the home, and practical assistance provided by informal carers. The use of SSD/SWD community and hospital social workers represented an average weekly cost of £5.28 (high cost estimate) and £3.52 (low cost estimate) per respondent.

Practical goods and services consist of a range of practical local authority, health service and voluntary agency assistance used by people with HIV infection or AIDS as a consequence of their HIV status. The goods and services used and costed were meals in the home, an occupational therapy service, grants for specific purchases from voluntary agencies or the SSD/ health authority, equipment for the home (eg, washing machines, cookers) and home adaptions (eg, central heating installed) supplied by statutory or voluntary agencies, DSS mobility allowance, the SSD/SWD provision of travel cards or bus refunds, private services such as window cleaning and house removals and NHS/SSD provision of goods and services for the hearing, visual, speech and incontinence needs of the respondents. Despite the wide coverage of this package of social care/support most of these goods and services were provided on a one-off basis producing a relatively low cost, estimated at a weekly total of £4.87 per respondent (Table 5.12).

Health maintenance treatment and therapy consists of services such as meditation, massage and aromatherapy that were used by the respondents. These were provided by the private sector or through voluntary agencies. The high cost estimate of this service use was £3.41 per respondent per week, and £1.64 per respondent for the low cost estimate (Table 5.12). Part of this cost was borne by the respondents through payment of fees for particular services.

Practical and emotional support services used by the respondents since acquiring the virus represented the lowest average weekly cost of each of the packages of social care/support. This was a high cost estimate of £0.57 per respondent and a low cost estimate of £0.46 per respondent (Table 5.12). The costs included the estimated time of specialists involved in providing sexual, incontinence, diet and housing advice, and advice and support provided through the use of voluntary sector telephone helplines. Respondents had also received advice on work and financial matters from a variety of agencies since acquiring the virus. The costs of specialist time involved in the provision of this advice was not included in the total costs of the package of practical and emotional support as this use was less directly related to the respondents' HIV status than the other advice provided.

Table 5.13 highlights the variation in the average weekly costs (high cost estimate) of each package of social care. Home support accounts for 69 per cent of weekly costs for all respondents, rising to 78 per cent of weekly costs for respondents with AIDS.

Table 5.13 **High Cost Estimates of Weekly Costs per Respondents of the Packages of Social Care as a Proportion of Total Cost**

	HIV+	ARC	AIDS	Total
Home Support	56	64	78	69
Social Worker	16	12	8	12
Practical Goods and Services	14	14	8	11
Health Maintenance Therapy/ Treatment	11	9	6	8
Practical and Functional Support Services	3	1	1	1

Patterns of Service Use

Variations existed between the average costs of each service package according to the HIV+/ARC/AIDS status of the respondents. For each of the packages of social care/support the average cost per respondent of service use was greater for people with ARC and/or AIDS than for people who were HIV positive. The outcome was a wide variation between these respondents in the total weekly costs of the integrated packages of social care/support. Based on a high cost estimate, the respective weekly costs per respondent of service use were calculated as £105.84 for people with AIDS. £51.13 for people with ARC and £19.48 for people who were HIV positive (Table 5.12). The same pattern is evident from Table 5.12 for the low cost estimate with respective costs of £88.11, £39.53 and £17.41 per respondent.

These cost differences are due to the greater overall level of service use by each individual with ARC/AIDS. On average, the total package of social care/support for people with AIDS involved the use of a greater range of services by each individual than was the case for people with ARC. The low relative cost for people who were HIV positive was due to a less integrated package of service use, with each individual tending to use, at most, only one or a few services.

The average amount of home support from informal carers, volunteers and home helps that was used by people who were HIV positive was much less than that used by people with ARC or, in particular, people with AIDS. As Table 5.12 demonstrates, the weekly costs of the use of home support services by the respondents with ARC and AIDS was, on average, approximately three times and between seven and eight times greater respectively than the average cost of this service use by people who were HIV positive. For each group of respondents this represented the highest cost of any package at a weekly total of £82.78, £32.74, £10.87 per AIDS, ARC, HIV positive respondent respectively (based on a high cost estimate: this was £70.45, £26.07, £10.35 respectively for the low cost estimate). The findings suggest that home support becomes a more important component of the social care/support package as the HIV status of individuals change. Whilst 56 per cent of the total average costs of social care/support service use by HIV positive respondents consisted of home support inputs, the equivalent proportion of cost for people with ARC and AIDS was 64 per cent and 78 per cent respectively (high cost estimate basis) (Table 5.13).

The average costs of the use of services within each of the other packages of social care/support was greater for people with ARC or AIDS than for people who were HIV positive, albeit at lower levels of cost. The average costs of the use of practical goods and services was between two and four times greater for respondents with ARC or AIDS, at £7.02 and £8.59 per respondent respectively, compared to respondents who were HIV positive (£2.76 per respondent). This was based on high cost estimates which were very similar to the low cost estimates. In addition, there was a similar difference in the average costs of the use of social worker services and health maintenance treatment/therapy. On a high cost estimate, the average weekly cost of social work service use was £7.97 and £6.31 per AIDS and ARC respondent respectively, but only £3.17 per HIV positive respondent. The respective weekly costs for the health maintenance package were £5.94, £4.40 and £2.14 per AIDS, ARC and HIV positive respondent (based on a high cost estimate: the low cost estimate for people with ARC was particularly low at £1.11 per respondent).

Despite these cost differences the proportion of the total costs of social care/support that consisted of practical goods and services, social worker and health maintenance service use was lower for people with ARC/AIDS (see

Table 5.13). This suggests that such indirect support and treatment services are relatively less important as HIV status changes and incidence of illness increases. For people with ARC/AIDS direct practical support in the home from formal and informal carers represents a more significant cost. The use of practical advice regarding sex, diet, incontinence and housing and the use of helplines by people with AIDS (£0.56; high cost basis) demonstrated a lower average weekly cost compared to the cost of such service use by people with ARC, and was very similar relative to the cost of services received by people who were HIV positive (£0.66 and £0.54 per ARC and HIV positive respondent respectively; high cost basis). The costs of advice and emotional support received in this way were a relatively higher proportion of social care/support costs for people who were HIV positive.

In contrast to the high relative use of direct home support services (both emotional and practical) by people with ARC/AIDS, the cost pattern for services used by HIV positive respondents suggests a relatively greater desire to seek indirect small scale practical assistance, advice/support and alternative remedies prior to becoming ill or being unable to perform basic daily tasks (such as cooking, shopping and housework), for which home support is required.

Costs of Packages of Care per Service User

There were variations in the numbers of service users for each package of social care/support. The average weekly costs per service user are presented in this section (the term 'costs per service user' throughout the rest of this section refers only to the users of each individual service or care/support package discussed and not to the total number of service users—which is taken as the 181 respondents in the study). This cost is associated with the proportion of HIV positive, ARC, AIDS respondents who had used or were using particular services due to their having the virus, and the level of individual service use by these respondents.

Community and Hospital Based Social Work Services

The unit costs of community and hospital based social work services were represented by the estimated salary, on-costs and apportionment of overhead costs for an HIV specialist social worker (£17.34 per hour in London, £15.85 per hour elsewhere—this produced the high cost estimate) and for a non-specialist social worker (£13.41 per hour in London, £11.99 per hour elsewhere—this produced a low cost estimate).

A total of 52 respondents (29 per cent of all respondents) had used the services of community social workers due to their having the virus, whilst only 32 respondents (18 per cent of all respondents) had seen a hospital social worker. Respondents were asked how frequently they used the services of a social worker. Based on information from responses to the questionnaire the average length of session with a social worker was assumed to be 2.5 hours (0.5 hours of this was an estimate of the travel and administrative time incurred by the social worker). The frequency of use of the hospital and community social worker varied from once per week to use on a one-off basis.

Despite lower numbers using the hospital social work service, the level of use was on average greater than that of the community social work service. This resulted in a weekly cost for the use of hospital social work of £11.21 per service user, compared to £10.00 per service user for respondents using the services of a community social worker (high cost estimate). The respective low cost estimates were £8.30 and £7.13 per service user (Table 5.14).

Table 5.14   **Average Weekly Cost Per Service User of SSD/SWD Social Work Services, by HIV Status**

Social Work Service	HIV+	ARC	AIDS	Total
Community Social Worker				
No. of Service Users	24	17	11	52
% of Respondents	23	49	28	29
Low Cost Estimates (£ per week)	7.56	4.84	11.30	7.13
High Cost Estimates (£ per week)	9.89	6.42	15.96	10.00
Hospital Social Worker				
No. of Service Users	10	7	15	32
% of Respondents	9	20	38	18
Low Cost Estimates (£ per week)	8.04	12.12	7.28	8.30
High Cost Estimates (£ per week)	10.01	16.02	9.55	11.21

The evidence from the survey suggests that in general the use of hospital social work services increases as HIV status changes. While 38 per cent of respondents with AIDS (n=15) used hospital social work services, only 20 per cent of respondents with ARC (n=7) and only nine per cent of HIV positive respondents (n=10) did so. This pattern is likely to be associated with the relatively greater number of occasions that people with ARC or AIDS attend hospital (either as in-patients or on an out-patient basis). However, despite a greater proportionate use of hospital social work services by respondents with AIDS the average weekly cost of this service use was relatively low at £9.55 per service user (high cost estimate). In comparison, the weekly high cost estimate for people with ARC was £16.02 per service user and £10.01 per HIV positive service user.

There was also an inverse relationship between the proportion of HIV positive, ARC and AIDS respondents who used the services of a community social worker and the average cost of this service used by each user. Of respondents with ARC, 17 (49 per cent) had seen a community social worker at an average weekly cost of £6.42 per service user (high cost estimate). In contrast, only 23 per cent of HIV positive respondents (n=24) and 28 per cent of respondents with AIDS (n=11) had seen a community social worker due to having the virus. However, these respondents demonstrated a greater average level of service use resulting in a higher average weekly cost per HIV positive and AIDS service user of £9.98 and £15.96 respectively (high cost estimate).

Most of the respondents who had seen a hospital or community social worker had received practical advice and support, for example concerning benefits eligibility, help with rehousing, liaison with the voluntary sector. Of the respondents for whom the service received was known, only five used a social worker for emotional support of which none were people with AIDS.

Home Support Services

Three sets of unit costs were used to determine the weekly costs of home support services (ie, voluntary sector home care, SSD/SWD home help and informal care) that was being used by the respondents.

A high cost estimate assumed home support was provided by a paid worker. The hourly cost for a paid worker in an HIV specific voluntary agency was estimated at £14.13 in London and £12.84 elsewhere. This used the same salary rate and on-costs as was used for an HIV-specialist social worker but with a smaller apportionment of overheads to reflect the lesser central establishment costs incurred by voluntary agencies relative to a local authority. No non-HIV specific agencies provided home support for any of the respondents. The low cost estimate assumed that home support was provided by a trained volunteer (eg, volunteer buddy). The value of services provided by a volunteer used the hourly payment rate and on-costs for an SSD HIV specialist community care worker (and the non-specialist rate for overhead apportionment). This produced a unit cost of £8.95 per hour for HIV specific agency volunteers. Information was derived on respondents' frequency of use of voluntary agency home support, but not the time involved. For the costing it was assumed that each session of support involved three hours of the time of a voluntary agency worker/volunteer.

The high cost estimate for SSD/SWD domiciliary care was based on the unit cost of an HIV specialist community care worker, of £11.71 per hour in London (including the specialist worker apportionment for overheads). As no specialist home helps existed in the other study localities the low cost estimate was based on a unit cost of a generic home help of £5.22 per hour out of London and £6.31 in London (including on-costs and overhead apportionment). Respondents provided information on the frequency of visits from home helps and the time involved. This was used to determine the average costs of service use.

The value of each hour of informal care and support used by respondents was represented by the unit cost of a non-HIV specialist home help. This was £5.22 per hour (excluding London weighting). The costing was based on information derived from the respondents frequency of use of informal care for four practical tasks only (shopping, cooking, housework and laundry—these are tasks that a home help would be likely to assist with). It was assumed that each separate occasion on which informal care was provided involved three hours of the time of the carer.

Table 5.15 outlines the variations in the level of use and average costs per user of voluntary agency home support, SSD/SWD home care and informal care. The high cost estimates for voluntary agency home support, SSD/SWD home care and the single average weekly cost produced for informal care were similar at £56.08, £66.50 and £65.05 per service user respectively. This similarity is based on a higher relative unit cost of SSD/SWD and voluntary agency care (due mainly to on-costs and overhead apportionment for their workers).

Practical informal care was provided to a greater number of respondents on a more frequent basis than was the case for home support provided by the SSD/SWD or voluntary sector. Over a quarter, 28 per cent, of respondents (n=51) received help from informal carers for shopping, cooking, housework and/or laundry alone compared to seven per cent of respondents (n=11) using a home help and 15 per cent (n=27) who used services provided by a voluntary agency. The greater level of home care provided for each individual by informal carers becomes more apparent, in terms of average weekly costs of service use, if low cost estimates for Social Service and voluntary agency support are considered. The respective average weekly costs were £44.00 and £36.84 per service user, which is much less than the single estimate of £65.05 for informal care (Table 5.15).

Table 5.15 Average Weekly Costs per Service User of the Use of Home Support, by HIV Status

Home Support Service	HIV+	ARC	AIDS	Total
Voluntary Agency Home Support				
No. of Service Users	10	9	8	27
% of Respondents	9	26	20	15
Low Cost Estimate (£ per week)	11.50	26.01	84.62	36.84
High Cost Estimate (£ per week)	17.05	39.61	189.30	56.08
SSD/SWD Domicilary Care				
No. of Service Users	1	3	7	11
% of Respondents	—	9	18	7
Low Cost Estimate (£ per week)	13.06	43.11	48.86	44.00
High Cost Estimate (£ per week)	13.06	80.00	68.29	66.50
Informal Care[1]				
No. of Service Users	19	11	21	51
% of Respondents	18	31	53	28
Cost Estimate (£ per week)	51.03	49.92	85.66	65.05

[1] Covers only assistance with four basic tasks—cooking, shopping, housework and laundry. In total 44, 16 and 21 respondents, HIV+, ARC and AIDS respectively received 'informal care'.

Table 5.15 demonstrates that a relatively intensive level of support was provided by voluntary agencies for some of the respondents with AIDS. Of respondents with AIDS 20 per cent (n=8) received home support from a voluntary agency costing on average £189.30 per week (high cost estimate, £84.62 per service user on a low cost estimate). This cost was related to the priority use of the time of buddies and other specially trained volunteers (eg, from THT, Frontliners) being given to providing emotional and practical support for people with AIDS. In contrast 26 per cent of respondents with ARC (n=9) and only nine per cent of respondents who were HIV positive (n=10) used voluntary sector home support of an average weekly cost of £39.61 and £17.05 per service user respectively (based on a high cost estimate—the low cost estimates were £26.01 and £11.50). SSD/SWD home care was used by very few respondents; by only one user who was HIV positive, three with ARC and seven with AIDS.

The need for assistance with cooking, shopping, housework and laundry increases as disability increases. The help of an informal carer in these tasks therefore tends to be more time consuming for people with ARC or AIDS. Support from partners, friends and family, if available, can generally be provided on a more flexible basis than statutory home care or even help from a voluntary agency. In many cases it is the first help that people will turn to, using other support only when informal care is not available or needs supplementing. In the survey, the outcome was a high relative level of support for the respondents with AIDS, with 53 per cent of respondents with AIDS using informal care for the four main practical tasks considered (n=21) at an estimated average weekly cost of £85.66 per service user (Table 5.15). The use of informal care by respondents with ARC and those who were HIV positive only was high compared to other forms of home support. The respective average weekly costs for informal help that was received by 31 per cent of ARC (n=11) and 18 per cent of HIV positive (n=19) respondents were £49.92 and £51.03 per service user (Table 5.15).

The costs of ad hoc advice and emotional support received by informal carers from statutory and voluntary sector specialists (eg, HIV counsellors, health advisers, THT counsellors) was estimated. The carers of 10 people who were HIV positive (nine per cent), seven people with ARC (20 per cent) and 10 people with AIDS (25 per cent) had received advice/support representing respective average weekly costs of £0.24, £0.35 and £0.31 per service user.

Practical Goods and Services

The cost of the use of a range of practical goods and services were assessed.

Only five respondents (three per cent of all respondents) had received a meals in the home service from the SSD/SWD (one person who was HIV positive had meals provided by a voluntary agency). Three respondents used a meals service on one occasion each week, and one person with ARC had been provided with a meal on five days each week. It was assumed that the provision of each meal involved on average an hour of the time of a member of staff, costed at £6.31 in London and £5.22 elsewhere, and the costs of the food (£1.00 per meal in London, £0.75 per meal elsewhere).

Table 5.16   **Average Weekly Cost per Service User of a Meals Service, by HIV Statis**

Meals Service	HIV+	ARC	AIDS	Total
No. of service users	1	1	3	5
% of respondents	—	3	8	3
Cost estimate (£ per week)	5.76	36.56	5.24	11.65

Table 5.16 demonstrates an average weekly cost of £11.65 per meals service user, with average costs per HIV positive, ARC and AIDS service user of £5.76 (1 person), £36.56 (1 person) and £5.24 (3 people) respectively.

Nine respondents used the services of an SSD/SWD occupational therapist (5 per cent of all respondents). This consisted of three people who were HIV positive and six people with AIDS (Table 5.17). Details were obtained of mobility devices and other equipment received subsequent to assessment by an OT. It was assumed that respondents received one OT assessment session each lasting four hours with an additional hour incurred by the OT in travel and administration (this estimate was drawn from responses on the questionnaire for Occupational Therapists).

Table 5.17   **Average Weekly Cost per Service User of SSD/SWD Occupational Therapy Services, by HIV Status**

Occupational Therapy Service	HIV+	ARC	AIDS	Total
No. of service users	3	—	6	9
% of respondents	3	—	15	5
Low cost estimate (£ per week)	1.45	—	3.77	3.03
High cost estimate (£ per week)	1.55	—	4.30	3.38

A high cost estimate was produced based on the use of an HIV specialist OT in London (£16.93 per hour—salary, on-costs and an overhead costs apportionment). The low cost estimate used the unit costs of a non specialist OT (£13.78 per hour in London, £12.37 per hour elsewhere—no HIV specialist OTs were employed in any of the study localities except in London). Equipment provided was costed at its manufacturer's price (this included walking supports, entry phone, bath rails, raised toilet seat). The current costs of this equipment was estimated on an annual basis over its useful life (estimated at five years) and discounted (using a 5 per cent discount rate) to reflect the additional cost incurred in not being able to use this money for other purposes during this time (eg, to invest in an interest bearing account).

The use of an OT involved assessment and equipment recommendation. The average weekly cost this was estimated at £3.38 per service user (on a high cost basis, £3.03 per service user on a low cost basis, Table 5.17). By HIV status, this was £1.55 per HIV positive service user and £4.30 per AIDS service user (reflecting the greater amount and cost of equipment received by the respondents with AIDS).

The costs of travel cards, taxi cards, annual bus passes and bus fare refunds provided to respondents by an SSD/SWD was based on an estimated annual cost per pass/card of £170.00, or an average of £3.27 per week. This was the average cost of passes/cards supplied to people with HIV-AIDS in 1989/90 by Kensington and Chelsea SSD (who had a special budget for this). The mobility and travel difficulties faced by people with ARC/AIDS resulted in 49 per cent of respondents with ARC (n=17) and 58 per cent of respondents with AIDS (n=23) having received some form of travel card/ assistance. In contrast, only eight per cent of respondents who were HIV positive (n=9) received such assistance.

There were 18 respondents in receipt of mobility allowance from the DSS (10 per cent of all respondents) which in 1989/90 was £23.05 per week. Mobility allowance was received by 28 per cent of respondents with AIDS (n=11), nine per cent of respondents with ARC (n=3) and four per cent of respondents who were HIV positive (n=4).

Health service specialists were seen by different respondents for hearing and visual needs. As Table 5.18 demonstrates this involved 10 respondents (four who were HIV positive, three with ARC and three with AIDS). In

Table 5.18   **Average Weekly Cost per Service User of Services for Hearing/Visual/ Incontinence Problems, by HIV Status**

Services for Hearing/Visual/ Incontinence Problems	HIV+	ARC	AIDS	Total
No. of service users	4	4	4	12
% of respondents	4	11	10	7
Cost estimate (£ per week)	1.05	0.55	0.79	0.79

addition, one person with ARC and one person with AIDS received sheets and pads from the SSD for bowel disorder problems. Visits to an eye consultant were costed at £21.09 per hour (salary, on-costs and overheads) in London (no such visits were made outside of London), using an estimate of 1.5 hours per consultation. The costs of special spectacles and sheets/pads provided were based on estimated manufacturers' prices. The average weekly cost of this service use by the 12 respondents (seven per cent of all respondents) was estimated at £0.79 per service user, with costs of £0.79, £0.55 and £1.05 per AIDS, ARC and HIV positive respondents respectively (Table 5.18).

The voluntary sector were involved in providing money for the purchase of practical goods and services for a third of the respondents (n=56, 31 per cent of all respondents). Agencies such as CRUSAID, Body Positive, Scottish AIDS Monitor and ACET provided grants, eg, for furnishing accommodation, a holiday, gas/electricity bills, clothes. The actual grant involved was recorded by respondents. In total this represented a weekly cost (over one year) of £4.12 per service user (Table 5.19). This average cost was highest for the provision made to people with AIDS, at £5.44 per service user (43 per cent of respondents with AIDS received special grants, n=17). The average weekly cost for the 46 per cent of respondents with ARC who received special grants (n=16) was less at £3.27 per service user. Grants were received by 22 per cent of respondents who were HIV positive (n=23) representing an average weekly cost of £3.75 per service user (Table 5.19).

Table 5.19   **Average Weekly Cost per Service User of Grants Provided by Voluntary Agencies for the Purchase of Practical Goods and Services, by HIV Status**

Voluntary Agency Grants	HIV+	ARC	AIDS	Total
No. of service users	23	16	17	56
% of respondents	22	46	43	31
Cost estimate (£ per week)	3.75	3.27	5.44	4.12

Private services such as house removals, window cleaning, house cleaning, gardening were used by eight per cent of respondents (n=14) related to their having the virus. The assumption is that these services would not have been required if the respondent had not acquired HIV infection (ie, the individual would not have undertaken the activity, such as moving house, or would have done it themselves, such as gardening). The level of use varied, generally being once a week or once per month, or on a one-off basis (for example, moving house). The cost of this service use was borne by the respondent. There was no particular pattern to this service use according to HIV status, with eight per cent of respondents with AIDS (n=3), 11 per cent of respondents with ARC (n=4) and seven per cent of respondents who were HIV positive (n=7) using private services at respective average weekly costs of £8.92, £3.68 and £4.07 per service user (Table 5.20). The total average weekly cost amounted to £5.00 per service user.

Table 5.20 **Average Weekly Cost Per Service User of Practical Private Sector Services by, HIV Status**

Practical Private Services	HIV+	ARC	AIDS	Total
No. of service users	7	4	3	14
% of respondents	7	11	8	8
Cost estimate (£ per week)	4.07	3.68	8.92	5.00

A total of 27 respondents (15 per cent of all respondents) had acquired home equipment, appliances or adaptions such as washing machines, cookers, bedding and central heating from a voluntary agency, the SSD/SWD or health authority. Based on estimated manufacturers' prices for such equipment, the average weekly cost estimated was £0.99 per service user (based on a seven year useful life for equipment and a five per cent discount rate). There was very little difference in average weekly cost according to HIV status with a range of £0.97 to £1.00 per service user (Table 5.21).

Table 5.21 **Average Weekly Cost per Service User of Home Equipment, Applicances and Adaptions Provided, by HIV Status**

Home Equipment/Appliances/ Adaptions	HIV+	ARC	AIDS	Total
No. of service users	9	9	9	27
% of Respondents	8	26	23	15
Cost estimate (£ per week)	0.97	0.99	1.00	0.99

Overall, the main users of practical goods and services (in terms of proportion of respondents and average cost) were the respondents with AIDS and, slightly less, the respondents with ARC. As Table 5.22 demonstrates, 55 per cent of respondents with ARC/AIDS (n=41) used one or more services contained within the practical goods and services package, compared to just 24 per cent of HIV positive respondents (n=25). The average weekly cost of the practical support was £15.62 per AIDS service user, but only £12.94 and £11.70 per ARC and HIV positive service user respectively (Table 5.22).

Table 5.22   **Average Weekly Cost per Service User of the Use of Services within the Practical Goods and Services Package, by HIV Status**

Practical Goods and Services	HIV+	ARC	AIDS	Total
No. of service users	25	19	22	66
% of respondents	24	54	55	36
Low cost est. (£ per week)	11.70	12.94	15.47	13.31
High cost est. (£ per week)	11.71	12.94	15.62	13.37

Health Maintenance Therapy and Treatment

The respondents provided details of the level of use and payments for health maintenance services such as massage, aromatherapy and visualisation. No information was collected on the frequency of use of special therapy/treatment provided free to the respondent by a voluntary agency. For those respondents paying for special therapy treatment, a high cost estimate was based on the assumption that service use (costed at price per session in the private sector) was weekly for three quarters of the year (39 weeks). The low cost estimate assumed the service was used on only four occasions during one year. Average weekly costs were based on the estimate of annual cost of each service user divided by 52 weeks.

As Table 5.23 demonstrates, over one third of respondents (n=61) had made use of special therapy/treatment due to their having the virus. For 35

Table 5.23   **Average Weekly Cost per Service User of the use of Health Maintenance Therapy/Treatment Services, by HIV Status**

Therapy/Treatment Service	HIV+	ARC	AIDS	Total
No. of service users	28	13	20	61
% of respondents	26	37	50	34
Low cost est. (£ per week)	5.34	2.99	5.50	4.87
High cost est. (£ per week)	8.10	11.85	11.88	10.11

respondents (19 per cent of all respondents) this was provided privately (and paid for by the respondent). Of the 26 respondents who received such services through a voluntary agency, nine paid a fee. In total, the average weekly cost of the use of health maintenance therapy/treatment ranged from £4.87 per service user (low cost estimate) to £10.11 per service user (high cost estimate).

The proportion of people using such services differed according to HIV status. Only 26 per cent of people who were HIV positive (n=28) used special therapies/treatments, compared to 37 per cent of respondents with ARC (n=13) and 50 per cent of respondents with AIDS (n=20). The level of private service use varied from a session per week for a set period or indefinitely, to one-off sessions, with a specialist. Based on the high cost estimate the respondents with ARC/AIDS demonstrated highest average weekly costs of special service use at £11.85/£11.88 per service user respectively (Table 5.23). For HIV positive service users the average weekly high cost estimate was lower at £8.10. However, whilst the findings suggest that the probability of people with ARC/AIDS using special therapies/treatments is greater than such use by people who are HIV positive only, the low cost estimate of service use demonstrated no systematic difference in average weekly costs according to HIV status. This cost was £5.34, £2.99 and £5.50 per HIV positive, ARC and AIDS service user respectively (Table 5.23).

Practical and Emotional Support Services

Advice regarding diet, sex life, bowel disorders and housing were obtained by respondents from a range of medical, local authority and voluntary agency sources. It was assumed this involved, on average, one hour of the time of a paid specialist (eg, dietician, hospital doctor, consultant, urologist, welfare officer, social worker, voluntary agency worker) with unit cost based on their hourly salary, direct on-costs and overhead apportionment (low rate). The use of voluntary agency helplines was costed assuming each call was received by an HIV specialist volunteer (unit cost of £8.95 per hour), made at the local cheap call rate and lasting for 30 minutes (high cost estimate producing a cost per call of £4.75) or 10 minutes (low cost estimate producing a cost per call of £1.58).

Over three quarters, 77 per cent, of all respondents (n=139) had received advice on diet, sex life, bowel disorders, housing or had used a helpline. This represented a low cost element of support for people with HIV infection, with a range for the average weekly cost of this service use of £0.47 (low cost estimate) to £0.74 (high cost estimate) per service user (Table 5.24).

A relatively large proportion of people diagnosed with ARC used specific advice/helpline services (89 per cent of respondents, n=31), compared to 75 per cent of respondents with AIDS (n=30) and 74 per cent of HIV positive respondents (n=78). In addition, a greater relative proportion of respondents with ARC used helpline services alone (43 per cent compared to 29 per cent and 33 per cent of HIV+/AIDS respondents). Of those using helpline services, the respondents who were HIV positive demonstrated highest levels of use with an average of seven calls, compared to only four calls per ARC/ AIDS service users. These findings suggest that people with HIV infection obtain emotional support and specific advice about various aspects of living with the virus before they develop AIDS. Indeed, this may be associated with a relatively lower use of practical home support or other special goods and services.

Table 5.24   **Average Weekly Cost per Service User of Use of Specific Advice Services/ Telephone Helplines, by HIV Status**

Advice on Diet, Sex Life, Incontinence, Housing and Helpline Services	**HIV+**	**ARC**	**AIDS**	**Total**
Helpline Services				
No. of service users	34	15	13	62
% of respondents	29	43	33	34
Average no. of calls per service user	7	4	4	5
Low cost est. (£ per week)	0.18	0.11	0.11	0.15
High cost est. (£ per week)	0.54	0.33	0.33	0.44
All helpline/specific advice services				
No. of service users	78	31	30	139
% of respondents	74	89	75	77
Low cost est. (£ per week)	0.57	0.63	0.65	0.47
High cost est. (£ per week)	0.73	0.74	0.75	0.74

There was virtually no difference in the average costs of the use of specific advice/helpline services according to respondent's HIV status (£0.73–£0.75 per service user-high cost estimate, see Table 5.24). The high cost estimate for helpline service use only was £0.54, £0.33, £0.33 per HIV positive, ARC and AIDS service user respectively (Table 5.24).

Average Weekly Costs of Packages of Care

Table 5.25 provides a summary of the average weekly costs of the use by respondents of services grouped within each of the packages of social care/support. In broad terms, the findings suggest a high relative level of use and hence cost of practical support and services (such as home assistance and equipment/services that assist daily living) by respondents with AIDS and, less so, respondents with ARC. Although practical services represented a major cost element of service use by respondents with HIV only, this was

Table 5.25   **Summary of Average Costs per Service User for Each Package of Social Care/Support, by HIV Status**

Social Care/Support Packages	Average costs (£ per week)			
	HIV+	ARC	AIDS	Total
Social Worker	(n=32)	(n=23)	(n=25)	(n=80)
Low cost estimate	5.98	5.97	7.08	6.32
High cost estimate	9.92	9.33	11.42	10.22
Home Support				
Voluntary and SSD/SWD	(n=11)	(n=9)	(n=9)	(n=29)
Low cost estimate	11.64	40.38	113.22	49.29
High cost estimate	16.69	66.28	168.00	74.86
Informal Care	(n=19)	(n=11)	(n=21)	(n=51)
Low cost estimate	51.03	44.92	85.66	66.05
Practical Goods and Services	(n=25)	(n=19)	(n=22)	(n=66)
Low cost estimate	11.70	12.96	15.47	13.31
High cost estimate	11.71	12.96	15.62	13.37
Health Maintenance Therapy/ Treatment	(n=28)	(n=13)	(n=20)	(n=61)
Low cost estimate	5.34	2.99	5.50	4.87
High cost estimate	8.10	11.85	11.88	10.11
Advice/Emotional Support	(n=78)	(n=31)	(n=30)	(n=139)
Low cost estimate	0.57	0.63	0.65	0.47
High cost estimate	0.73	0.74	0.75	0.74

less than for people with AIDS. The greater relative use of advice and help-line services by HIV positive and ARC respondents may be inversely related to the practical, material and physical support they receive from informal carers, voluntary agencies and the SSD/SWD.

Average Costs According to Source of Service Provision

The services used by respondents were supplied from a variety of sources. The average cost of the use of services provided by each of the voluntary, statutory (ie, local authority/NHS/other) and private sectors have been determined and are presented in Table 5.26 (the average costs per service user for informal care are included in Tables 5.15 and 5.25). The costs of all private sector services used were incurred by the respondents, whilst most of the costs for voluntary/statutory services were met by the service provider. This costing (as with that for each service package) did not include an assessment of the personal time and money costs incurred by respondents' use of services, apart from fees paid to cover service charges.

Table 5.26   **Average Weekly Costs Per Service User of Voluntary, Statutory and Private Sector Social Care/Support Services, by HIV Status**

Service Provider	HIV+	ARC	AIDS	Total
Voluntary Sector				
No. of service users	55	28	25	108
% of respondents	52	80	63	60
Low cost est. (£ per week)	4.29	12.61	32.14	12.90
High cost est. (£ per week)	6.94	19.94	51.63	20.66
Statutory Sector[1]				
No. of service users	51	28	10	89
% of respondents	48	80	25	49
Low cost est. (£ per week)	9.23	16.03	80.80	19.08
High cost est. (£ per week)	10.68	23.21	103.00	25.89
Private Sector[2]				
No. of service users	21	10	12	43
% of respondents	20	29	30	24
Cost est. (£ per week)	8.03	3.22	9.50	7.28

[1] Local authority/NHS/DSS

[2] Cost met by respondents using private services

Variations existed in the pattern of costs according to the source of supply for the services used. Overall, there was a greater proportion of respondents using the services of the voluntary sector (60 per cent of respondents, n=108) compared to the use of statutory or private sector services (49 per cent of respondents, n=89, and 24 per cent of respondents, n=43, respectively). However, the findings suggest that the use of voluntary agency services represents a lower cost option for services in which a choice of service provider exists. The estimated average weekly cost of voluntary agency service use was £12.90 (low cost estimate) to £20.66 (high cost estimate) per voluntary sector service user, compared with an average cost for statutory service use of £19.08 to £25.89 per service user. The charges that were levied for the private sector operated as a disincentive to their use as the costs were generally met by the respondents. This resulted in a relatively low average weekly cost per private sector service user of £7.28.

A relatively high proportion of respondents with ARC used services provided by the voluntary or statutory sector, but at an average weekly cost below that of the service use of respondents with AIDS (Table 5.26). A total of 80 per cent (n=56) of respondents with ARC used voluntary and statutory services at an average weekly cost per service user of £12.61 to £19.94 (voluntary sector services) and £16.03 to £23.21 (statutory sector services). In contrast, whilst only 63 per cent (n=25) and 25 per cent (n=10) of respondents with AIDS used voluntary and statutory services respectively, this represented a relatively high average weekly cost per service user of £32.14 to £51.63 (voluntary sector services) and £80.80 to £103.00 (statutory sector services).

Amongst the highest average weekly costs per service user were those for the use of informal care (Table 5.25). This demonstrates the important cost associated with the role of informal care in the practical (and emotional) support of people with HIV infection, in particular for people with AIDS. In the survey the respondents with AIDS demonstrated the highest average weekly cost for informal care of £85.66 per service user.

The respondents who were HIV positive demonstrated the lowest average weekly costs for the use of voluntary services at £4.29 to £6.94 per service user, and for the use of statutory sector services at £9.23 to £10.68 per service user. However, the proportion of HIV positive respondents using these services, at 52 per cent for voluntary agency service use (n=55) and 48 per cent for statutory sector service use (n=51), was only slightly below that for the respondents with AIDS. It is likely that many of the respondents who were HIV positive only, relative to people with ARC/AIDS, were not given priority (or were not eligible) for social care/support services provided by statutory or voluntary agencies. The high relative cost of £8.03 per HIV positive service user for the use of private services (by 20 per cent of HIV positive respondents) suggests some of these respondents purchased services to supplement (or substitute for) the use of statutory and voluntary services.

5.5 National Cost Estimates

The cost estimates shown in Table 5.27 can be used to produce a rough estimate of the aggregate costs of the potential demand for HIV-AIDS related social care in the UK based on a total of 1,623 people with AIDS at the end of June 1990. This produces a national cost of service demand by people with AIDS of £143,000–£172,000 per week or £7.4 million to £8.9 million over one year (ie, weekly cost multiplied by 52 weeks). Similarly, there were 14,090 people who were known to be HIV positive only in June 1990. Using the average cost estimates produced a total potential demand cost of providing social care for people who are known to be HIV positive for the UK of £245,000 to £275,000 per week or £12.7 million to £14.3 million over one year. If it is assumed that 14,090 HIV+ people also includes people with ARC, the total national cost of providing social care to people who are HIV positive, have ARC or AIDS is estimated at £388,000 to £447,000 per week or £20.1 million to £23.2 million per year.

These figures provide a crude estimate of the true cost of providing the same level of service nationally as has been received by the respondents in the survey from the five areas in which the demand for social care for people with HIV-AIDS is already being established.

Table 5.27   **Average and Aggregate[1] Cost of Demand**

Average/Aggregate Costs		Low Cost Estimate	High Cost Estimate
Average cost of service use per person with AIDS	—£s per week	88.11	105.84
Aggregate costs of service use by people with AIDS[2]	—£s per week —£s per year	143,000 7.4 million	172,000 8.9 million
Average cost of service use per person HIV+ only[3]	—£s per week	17.41	19.41
Aggregate costs of service use by people HIV+ only[4]	—£s per week —£s per year	245,000 12.7 million	275,000 14.3 million
Total aggregate cost of service use by people HIV+, with ARC or AIDS[5]	—£s per week —£s per year	388,000 20.1 million	447,000 23.2 million

[1] The aggregate cost estimates represent the cost of providing the same level of service nationally as has been received by the respondents in the five study areas.

[2] Based on a figure of 1623 people alive with AIDS as of June 1990 (calculated by CDSC/CD(S)U).

[3] Based on a figure of 14,090 people known to be HIV+ as of June 1990 (calculated by CDSC/CD(S)U).

[4] The HIV+ cost estimates have used the social care package data and assumed the cost of HIV+ and ARC social care packages are the same. This assumption is made because it is not possible to distinguish HIV+ and ARC cases in national data provided by CDSC/CD(S)U although it is, from the Hull-York survey, possible to distinguish service cost differences for these groups.

[5] Based on the total number of people known to be HIV+, have ARC or alive with AIDS (ie, 14,090 + 1,623 = 15,713).

Printed in the United Kingdom
Dd294539 2/93 C20 G531 10